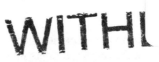

LIVERPOOL L2 2ER
TEL. 0151 231 4022

**Palliative care
in the home**

LIVERPOOL JMU LIBRARY

3 1111 01014 9779

Oxford University Press makes no representation, express or implied, that the drug dosages in this book are correct. Readers must therefore always check the product information and clinical procedures with the most up-to-date published product information and data sheets provided by the manufacturers and the most recent codes of conduct and safety regulations. The authors and the publishers do not accept any responsibility or legal liability for any errors in the text or for the misuse or misapplication of material in this work.

Palliative care in the home

Derek Doyle OBE, D.Sc., FRCSEd, FRCPEd, FRCP Lond., FRCGP
Vice-President of the National Council for Hospice and Specialist Palliative Care Services
President Emeritus of the International Hospice Institute and College
Formerly Medical Director, St. Columba's Hospice Edinburgh

David Jeffrey, MA, FRCPEd, MRCGP
Macmillan Lead Palliative Care Consultant
3 Counties Cancer Centre, Cheltenham General Hospital
Honorary Senior Lecturer in Palliative Medicine, University of Bristol

Foreword by
Sir Kenneth Calman, KCB, FRSE
Vice-Chancellor, University of Durham
Formerly Chief Medical Officer of England and Scotland

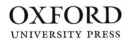

OXFORD
UNIVERSITY PRESS

OXFORD
UNIVERSITY PRESS

Great Clarendon Street, Oxford OX2 6DP

Oxford University Press is a department of the University of Oxford. It furthers the University's objective of excellence in research, scholarship, and education by publishing worldwide in

Oxford New York

Athens Auckland Bangkok Bogotá Buenos Aires Calcutta Cape Town Chennai Dar es Salaam Delhi Florence Hong Kong Istanbul Karachi Kuala Lumpur Madrid Melbourne Mexico City Mumbai Nairobi Paris São Paulo Singapore Taipei Tokyo Toronto Warsaw

with associated companies in Berlin Ibadan

Oxford is a registered trade mark of Oxford University Press in the UK and in certain other countries

Published in the United States by Oxford University Press Inc., New York

© Oxford University Press 2000

The moral rights of the author have been asserted

Database right Oxford University Press (maker)

Previously published as *Domicillary Palliative Care (1994)*

All rights reserved. No part of this publication may be reproduced, stored in a retrieval system, or transmitted, in any form or by any means, without the prior permission in writing of Oxford University Press, or as expressly permitted by law, or under terms agreed with the appropriate reprographics rights organization. Enquiries concerning reproduction outside the scope of the above should be sent to the Rights Department, Oxford University Press, at the address above

You must not circulate this book in any other binding or cover and you must impose this same condition on any acquirer

British Library Cataloguing in Publication Data
Data available

Library of Congress Cataloguing in Publication Data
1 3 5 7 9 10 8 6 4 2

ISBN 0-19-2632272 (Pbk)

Typeset in Minion by Florence Production Ltd
Printed in Great Britain on acid-free paper
by Biddles Ltd, Guildford & King's Lynn

Foreword

Sir Kenneth Calman, KCB, FRSE

Over the last few years much has changed in clinical practice and palliative care is no exception. This book on palliative care, dealing with patient problems in the home, reflects these changes. First, there has been a significant increase in patient knowledge and expectations. This must be a good thing, and indeed is to be encouraged. However, it does have consequences. Patients are much more knowledgeable and expect more from their doctor and the primary care team. The views of the patient are paramount and need to be reflected in the quality of the service provided.

Second, there has been a welcome return towards a broader, more holistic approach to care for the patient which can be delivered close to home. The chapters in this volume on spiritual aspects of care and on the ethical problems that arise are very relevant to this. Once again we should welcome this broader view of clinical practice. It is also reflected in the need for multidisciplinary care, respecting and encouraging the skills of a wide range of healthcare professionals. They add so much to the improvements in quality of life, which can now be achieved.

The third aspect is the increasing emphasis on clinical skills, of diagnosis and management. Listening to patients remains at the heart of what doctors do, together with giving practical advice and help where it is required. The chapters on emergencies in palliative care and some of the more practical aspects of palliative care are well covered, particularly in the appendices. Thus the reference to what one might carry in the doctor's bag is particularly helpful.

This book is a guide, it sets direction, gives advice on making decisions and on management. It emphasizes the importance of dealing with the needs of individual patients and how best to improve quality of life. This book is for every member of the primary care team and, if used wisely, will help to improve the quality of care provided.

We dedicate this book to
Bethia and Pru

Preface

Providing good palliative care is always challenging but nowhere more so than in the patient's home. Not only is it always challenging—it is also rewarding. It is our hope that this book will help doctors and nurses offering palliative care in the home to get the maximum professional satisfaction out of this responsibility because they know they are offering the best care possible.

Perhaps a few words about the title of the book would be in order. Very deliberately we have chosen the now well-established term 'palliative care' in preference to terminal care, hospice care, care of the dying, or similar descriptions. We have done so because it is now a universally accepted term in spite of the ambiguity inherent in it. The care we shall describe is much more than the care needed in the last days of life, although that is described in a separate chapter in the book. In some respects it may resemble the care offered in hospices, but it is more than that. It focuses on the special, sometimes the unique, problems faced in a person's home, often quite different from many encountered in a hospice.

This book has evolved from another one, said to have been much appreciated and now translated into several languages, entitled *Domiciliary palliative care*. However, some colleagues pointed out that the word domiciliary is not widely used or understood. No one could say that about the word home, meaning the patient's home or the home of a relative, or even a nursing home.

Who is the book written for? Once again we come up against problems of parlance. In the United Kingdom we would refer to the doctors caring for patients in their homes as general practitioners. In North America they are more usually called family physicians. In yet other parts of the world they are spoken of as primary care doctors or doctors of first contact. We appreciate that these different terms are not synonymous. General practice as we know it in the United Kingdom only exists there and in a few other places, but in most countries with reasonably well-developed healthcare systems there are doctors, whatever they are termed, who see people in or near their homes rather than in hospitals. This book is written with them all in mind. In such systems there are nurses—again their titles vary greatly—who assist in the care of the person at home, nurses who work closely with the doctor, and are often based in the same building as the doctor and his or her partners. Such nurses are, like the doctor, indispensable. This book is also for them. Throughout the book we have tried to make our text understandable and useful for colleagues not working in the United Kingdom, knowing how much people increasingly look to us for help in providing high-quality palliative care.

One glance at the book will show that it is not a reference book, a textbook fit for the library shelf. It does not purport to be that but it is certainly written for quick reference, either in the doctor's consulting room or more likely on his/her return from a person's home. Perhaps the description coined by one of our colleagues is the most apt—'a recipe book rather than a reference book'. For those who want to delve deeper, or even to ensure that what is suggested is evidence-based, the major texts on the subject are listed in an appendix.

Readers will soon appreciate that everything is written with the patient's home in mind, not the local hospice or specialist palliative care unit. We describe the problems as they will present there and suggest appropriate treatment. The specialist treatment that might be available in a hospital or palliative care unit is mentioned only so that the doctor and nurse working in the home know when to refer or consult, and what their patient might receive there.

Perhaps now is the time to introduce ourselves, the authors. What are our credentials and what has been our experience that we feel qualified to prepare such a book for colleagues? Both of us spent many years in general practice before eventually moving into careers in specialist palliative medicine. Not only did we work as general practioners, we also taught general practice at university level, taught GP registrars, and did research in general practice. One of us (D.D.) has now retired, but as consultants in palliative medicine we were not locked into a hospital system but, on a daily basis, visited people in their own homes, talked to their doctors and nurses, and worked alongside oncologists, cardiologists, and others. We feel we know what it is like working with patients in their homes. We have tried to keep up to date with recent developments and the many changes that have taken place in general practice. In addition, one of us has travelled extensively, lecturing and teaching, visiting patients in their own homes, and spending much time working with doctors in many of the countries of Europe and Australasia, as well as in countries as diverse as Saudi Arabia, Hong Kong, and South Korea. We are totally convinced that good palliative care should start in the home, whether or not the patient is eventually admitted to a hospital or specialist palliative care unit. Having said that, we are very conscious how difficult it is to deliver good palliative care and have dedicated a chapter to the challenges.

We have written the book very conscious of the many changes taking place in general practice, or its equivalent, around the world. Doctors and nurses feel that they are expected to care for more patients, in less time, against a background of rising public and political expectations. Their dedication to high-quality care is undiminished but they find themselves struggling to offer good care and at the same time coping with more bureaucracy and less understanding of their work and potential. As some have told us, they fear that the first group who might suffer are the most vulnerable, those who need palliative care.

One of the changes in recent years, and one to which we shall refer later, is the place to die in our modern society. In less than a century it has changed from the home to the hospital (or, for a few, the local hospice). What has not changed, however, is the ethical and professional imperative to provide the best care, for as long as possible, in the home, whether or not the person then stays there or is admitted for terminal care. As we shall discuss later, it is questionable whether doctors and nurses can much influence where a person dies, important as their input can be into the care at home.

Finally, we readily acknowledge that resources vary greatly between different countries and often within a country, indeed even between one suburb and another in a large city. There will inevitably be some readers who have to work in isolation and who will read of medical and nursing colleagues meeting to share their experiences, and will envy them. There will be others who cannot conceive of offering palliative care without the full range of opioids or access to the most sophisticated diagnostic facilities available.

May all our readers get as much challenge and as much pleasure out of offering palliative care as we have done in our clinical work and through writing this book.

Our thanks to nursing and medical colleagues for their advice and comments and to our patients and their families for teaching us so much.

Contents

1

The challenge of providing palliative care in the home

The goal of palliative care is to achieve the best quality of life for patients with incurable life-threatening diseases. Palliative care provides relief from pain and other distressing symptoms and offers a support system to help the family cope during the patient's illness and bereavement. Terminal care is that part of palliative care which takes place in the last days of life, when the aim is to enable the patient to die with dignity.

Although, in the Western world, one in four patients die from cancer, an individual general practitioner may only care for four or five patients dying at home from cancer each year. Some of the challenges facing primary care teams providing palliative care can be considered as follows:

♦ Communication

Palliative care is not a highly technological subject but it is highly sophisticated. It challenges doctors and nurses at a clinical and ethical level. The challenge may start from the time of diagnosis. In the community, patients present with ill-defined symptoms and there is often a delay before a diagnosis can be made. The doctor needs to acknowledge that there may have been a delay in diagnosis but this should not prevent a good trusting relationship with the patient.

When patients complain about delays in diagnosis, a common problem is that they felt that their initial symptoms were not taken seriously and were dismissed as trivial. Doctors can reduce the chance of complaints by adopting a less paternalistic attitude to patients presenting with vague symptoms.

There are communication challenges for the doctor in breaking the bad news, particularly when the cancer comes back and the situation becomes clearly palliative. The doctor needs to give the patient and relatives confidence that they will continue to be looked after and will not be abandoned merely because the cancer or life-threatening disease is no longer responsive to curative measures. Maintaining hope does not mean raising false hopes but rather setting realistic goals with the patient and family.

◆ Continuity

Continuity of care is difficult to organize but essential if high standards of palliative care are to be obtained. Patients and their families need to have access to doctors and nurses. They need to build a relationship with healthcare professionals, which is based on trust and confidence and allows both patients and relatives to discuss their most intimate fears.

With the changes in the organization of primary care within the United Kingdom, with the increasing use of co-operatives and less emphasis on home visiting, continuity becomes more difficult to provide.

Although in palliative care much can be done to relieve many symptoms and distress, not all suffering is relievable and there is the challenge of staying with and continuing to visit patients who have unrelieved suffering. When the dying process is prolonged, this can be particularly stressful to caring teams and relatives.

◆ Competency

General practitioners need to keep up to date with recent developments in pain and symptom control. One of the functions of multidisciplinary specialist palliative care teams is to act as a resource to provide up-to-date information to general practitioners. The professionals need to have confidence in each other to know that they can access specialist palliative care teams without fear of their care being criticized or of the specialist team taking over. One of the most effective ways of improving skills is by listening to and working with colleagues.

◆ Team working

Palliative care at home demands a multidisciplinary team approach. Specialist palliative care teams are well aware that patients and families want to be cared for by general practitioners and district nurses, and their role is to support them and to enable this to happen. General practitioners need to know what specialist resources are available within their area and when to involve specialist care. It is necessary also to explain to patients the role of specialist nurses to enable them to accept the help of specialist teams.

Different disciplines need to maintain clear channels of communication to acknowledge difficulties and to reach a consensus rather than perceiving one discipline as being critical of another.

◆ Ethical issues

There are a host of ethical dilemmas and problems that confront the primary care team, and these are heightened at the end of life. The choice of where to die is one of the most important and worrying for patients and families and needs to be explored sensitively. Like many decisions in this area, there must be opportunities for patients and relatives to change their minds as the course of the disease progresses and different problems arise.

To enable patients to have the maximum quality of life means respecting their autonomous choices. This places a requirement on the doctor to listen to the patient's and relative's view and to be aware that there is a requirement to seek informed, free, and negotiated consent when proposing any interventions or investigations.

We need to resist medical paternalism, particularly with patients who seem frail, vulnerable, and weak. On the other hand, some patients, once informed, want their professional team to make the medical decisions for them. This is perfectly acceptable provided that each time decisions are made these are checked out with the patient and the family and they are given an opportunity to state their views.

◆ Time

Providing palliative care at home requires an investment of time and this generates an ethical strain where such a resource is limited. The co-ordination of visits and the effective use of a telephone can improve care. The non-verbal behaviour of the doctor or nurse can create an impression that they are relaxed and are prepared to give plenty of time. Patients and their families are generally understanding of how busy doctors are. If community nurses are particularly hard-pressed and find difficulty giving enough time for listening to the patient and family, they may get effective support from community Macmillan nurses who may have more time available.

◆ Relatives and carers

Relatives and carers can present a different challenge. They may not voice their own needs, which are different from those of the patient. In particular, young children tend to be ignored by the professionals. Relatives often perceive that the patient's suffering is greater than professionals think. It is important to give time to the family to address their needs.

♦ Partnership

The key to palliative care is forming a partnership with patients, family, and professionals, where there is openness and honesty, and where patients are informed and respected. General practitioners and district nurses are in a unique and privileged position to provide this care. They have support from specialist teams to help them to continue to provide the highest standards of care at home.

2

Symptom palliation

General principles

By definition, by the time a person is receiving palliative care the diagnosis of their underlying disease has long been made and all potentially curative treatment has been given. That is not to say that much active treatment cannot still be helpful and, indeed, palliative care is itself active, sometimes energetic, and even modestly invasive. A high level of diagnostic suspicion must be maintained. We shall keep returning to this.

In recent years doctors have increasingly come to regard themselves primarily as diagnosticians. In palliative care their ability to diagnose is secondary to their ability to identify how the patient feels and to find means of relieving whatever suffering is reported or uncovered. Expressed another way—symptoms are now windows on to a patient's suffering of body or mind or spirit, not pointers to a primary diagnosis.

Several principles must be emphasized before specific symptoms are dealt with:

♦ Patients only report about 50 per cent of their symptoms

In fact they only mention the problems the doctor and nurses seem interested in even though other problems may trouble them more. For example, it is unusual for a doctor to be told of the symptoms of oral candidiasis. It is only when the doctor says 'Tell me every single thing, big or small, which is making life a misery for you at this time' that the patient mentions nightmares, sweating, changed taste perception, fears, and so much else.

♦ Patients mention different symptoms to nurses from those reported to doctors

Evidence suggests that nurses are told more about psychosocial problems while doctors hear more about physical problems. Whether this is because nurses often show more interest in the psychosocial is not clear. It does, however, underline the need for close collaboration between doctors and nurses if the whole picture is to be known.

LIVERPOOL
JOHN MOORES UNIVERSITY
AVRIL ROBARTS LRC
TITHEBARN STREET
LIVERPOOL L2 2ER
TEL. 0151 231 4022

♦ Patients stop reporting symptoms if no interest is shown in them or treatment fails

This is surprising when you see how much suffering they have. It is a reminder that terminally ill people are remarkably uncomplaining, almost stoical. It is not uncommon to meet one who has suffered pain for months and been kept on the same unhelpful analgesic. They say they reported the pain but no interest was shown and no attempt made to change the analgesic so they endured it bravely. A reminder that 'no pain reported' means just that—it might have been present but was no longer reported.

♦ Patients want to know/need to know the significance of each symptom

This is a feature almost unique to palliative care patients. For example, to the doctor dyspnoea is usually an index of respiratory, cardiac, or a blood disease, a reminder that an examination and possibly investigations need to be performed to come to a diagnosis. To the patient it suggests a frightening future of increasing breathlessness and diminishing activity, possible even a death from asphyxia. The palliative care patient who tells the doctor he is still breathless is not usually asking if he can be further investigated or if the doctor knows what is wrong with him, but is seeking reassurance that the doctor can help him and that he will not finally suffocate to death.

The person with steatorrhoea wants reassurance that his cancer is not being carried in the peculiar fatty stools. The one with dysphagia may know about his oesophageal carcinoma and why he has had radiotherapy, or a stent inserted, but each day wants reassurance that he will not choke or aspirate. Even more frequently, the patient who senses she is muddled or confused needs to be reassured that this is not the first sign of a mental illness. It always helps to say something like 'I realize you are worried about this. I'll explain everything to you but first, tell me what's on your mind, what's worrying you?'

♦ Patients mention physical problems before psychosocial ones before spiritual ones

So much is said about palliative care being holistic, concerned with physical, emotional, social, and spiritual problems, that some doctors and nurses expect patients to unburden all their problems, all the details of their illness, at once—a bolus of problems. They never do. Even with members of the primary care team, many of whom they will know well, they mention the physical issues and, as they are relieved, out come the emotional and social ones. It is sometimes far into their palliative care that they mention, or allude to, spiritual issues. It is as if we are being tested before being trusted with the difficult and delicate problems.

The importance of this is that we must never assume that because psychosocial and spiritual problems have not been aired they do not exist. They will come later, provided not too many professionals are involved in the care at any one time.

◆ Patients do not want a prescription for each symptom

Patients often say how much better they feel having reported some of the things troubling them. What they do not want, and are not expecting, is a prescription for everything they have mentioned—something for the pain, the dyspnoea, the anorexia, the constipation, the sweating, the insomnia, etc. What matters is that the doctor and nurses know of their suffering and, should the need ever arise, know how to deal with it. It is easy for the doctor to say 'you mentioned terrible sweating the last time I was in. Do you want anything for it or can you manage in the mean-time?'

We shall now look at some of the commonest symptoms.

Anorexia

Principal causes

◆ dry mouth (xerostomia), usually drug-induced

◆ oral candidiasis

◆ chronic constipation

◆ nausea and/or vomiting

◆ uninteresting, unimaginatively served food

◆ odours in the environment, even pleasant cooking smells

◆ anxiety state

◆ depressive state

◆ metabolic—hypercalcaemia, elevated liver function tests (LFTs), uraemia

◆ advancing disease.

It is uncommon for a palliative care patient to be anxious about loss of appetite, although there is usually much pleasure when it is restored. More usually, it is the relatives who report it. Like most people they regard a good appetite as a sign of health and also want to contribute to the patient's care through their cooking. In most cultures a meal taken with family or friends is a happy occasion, a time of sharing. Seeing a patient wanting to eat alone, taking little, and being uninterested in 'treats' is a stark reminder of mortality.

Management

1. Try to identify and remove the cause. It is nearly always possible to tidy up the medication, treat constipation, advise on cooking smells, and control candidiasis.

2. Explain that anorexia is partly caused by the cancer itself and is no reflection on the carer's ability to look after the patient. It is the absence of appetite which distinguishes the patient with advanced cancer from a person who is starving to death, who will experience hunger.

3. Advice on cooking and preparing suitable meals is both helpful and often surprising to relatives but the doctor must never give the impression that the disease is caused by poor diet or that the fatal outcome can be avoided by a change in diet.

4. Relatives need to be advised that the more ill the person is, the less they will eat in the evening and midday, and the largest meal (though still very modest) will be at breakfast. Small meals, offered frequently, on small plates, are better than standard helpings at traditional times. Relatives need to be told how fickle are the food likes and dislikes of the terminally ill; today's favourite will be refused tomorrow; yesterday's reject will be today's request. The special treat the wife goes out to buy in the morning will not be acceptable when she cooks it at midday. All very sad and trying for the carer, and difficult to understand and accept.

5. Terminally ill people like simple, almost nursery, foods such as porridge, ice cream, sorbet, yoghurt, cold custard, and cold stewed fruit. Coloured food is more tempting than tasty but drab food and carers should be advised to add colour in the form of dressing or yoghurt on ice cream, a sprig of parsley or mint on white fish, and a few drops of a liqueur on sorbet.

The temptation to suggest 'invalid' foods must be resisted. Most are not palatable and relatives are only further upset when the food which is said to restore energy and weight fails to do so.

There are only two drugs which have been shown to improve appetite, corticosteroids and megestrol acetate.

(a) Dexamethasone 2 milligrams morning and midday for 1 week followed by 2 milligrams in the morning only for the second week, then stop.

Continuing with steroids beyond 2–3 weeks is ineffective. If a second course is given the effect is usually less than in the first course.

(b) Megestrol acetate 160 milligrams three times daily for a minimum of 4 weeks both stimulates appetite and produces genuine weight gain, albeit for a short time. Little benefit is seen before 4 weeks. It has to be remembered that the tablets are large and very expensive.

When it is thought that the patient's prognosis is measurable in months, megestrol is the preferred drug. When it is much shorter but still long enough to enjoy boosted appetite, then prescribe the steroid.

Anxiety

Anxiety in the terminally ill person is understandable but need not be left unheeded or unrelieved. It is critically important to try to define the cause rather than treating empirically with anxiolytics.

Causes

- Fear of the unknown. The patient is unlikely to have had a life-threatening illness before, or to have felt so weak and increasingly dependent. He/she is unable to build on experience, remembering how they coped in the past.

- Fear of the possible, strange as this may sound. We are all much more affected than we like to admit by what we see and hear in the media, what we hear from relatives and friends. Increasing frailty impairs our critical objectivity so that we fall prey to primitive fears we might normally dismiss. Some examples will illustrate this. Terminally ill people dread psychiatric illness and even the most understandable moment of confusion or memory loss brings on their anxiety. They fear bleeding to death, hence their profound anxiety when they see a fleck of blood in a sputum mug or haematuria in the catheter bag. Conditioned as they might be to equate cancer with pain, even when they have no pain they expect it. Increasing dyspnoea, even when not disabling, is seen as a foretaste of asphyxia.

- Fear of the illness and its consequences. This cannot be overstated. The terminally ill person needs to know the meaning/cause of each new symptom as it affects him and not as the diagnostic feature it is to the doctor. This has been alluded to already and examples might include:

Dyspnoea: 'Am I likely to die of suffocation, fighting for breath?'

Haemoptysis: 'Will I bleed to death?'

Confusion at night or when wakening: 'Am I going mad?'

It is worth remembering that patients seem better able to recall horrific examples of suffering and complications amongst their friends and fellow patients they have seen in hospital than to remember the explanations and reassurances of their doctors.

- Fears of being a burden to others. Patients often express more anxiety about how their relatives are coping, and will cope after their death, than about themselves. The problem is compounded by the conspiracy of silence which so often surrounds the patient, each party protecting the other and neither feeling free to talk openly about their feelings.
- Drug-induced anxiety, for example when the sleep pattern is disrupted by dexamethasone given late in the day, when there is amnesia after midazolam, or when there is confusion as a result of excessive sedation.

Management

It is essential to explore possible causes before reaching for the prescription pad. This is one of those times when the sharing of knowledge and insights by doctor and nurse is so valuable.

The questions to be asked are:

1. Has every symptom been identified, explained and dealt with?

2. Has every fear been explored and all explanations by the professionals been consistent?

3. Are any of the symptoms or problems iatrogenic?

4. Is there a past history of anxiety, depression, drug or substance abuse, or psychiatric care?

Medication

- If anxiolytics are needed, start with short half-life benzodiazepines, e.g. lorazepam 1 milligram twice daily by mouth.
- If the oral route is not practical, use midazolam 1.25–2.5 milligrams subcutaneously.
- Use neuroleptics such as thioridazine and haloperidol when there are psychotic features such as delusions and hallucinations.

◆ The phenothiazines, chlorpromazine and methotrimeprazine, are useful when sedation is needed but their anticholinergic and hypotensive effects must be remembered.

◆ Tricyclic antidepressants are indicated when anxiety is a feature of a depressive state but their sedative and anticholinergic effects must be remembered.

Whatever drugs are being used there is a place for relaxation techniques, music therapy, visualization, guided imagery, and hypnosis, when employed by professionals fully trained in the procedure.

Ascites

Malignancy is the cause of 10 per cent of all cases of ascites and 15–50 per cent of patients with malignant disease will develop it. Thirty percent of women with ovarian carcinoma will have it at presentation and over 60 per cent by the time they die. It is associated with most of the malignancies seen in primary care including melanoma, mesothelioma, and myeloma.

Ascites is also a feature of other mortal illnesses leading to palliative care in the home, including liver disease with portal hypertension, cardiac failure, nephrotic syndrome, and, now on the increase again, tuberculosis.

In all patients it should be regarded as serious and worth palliating for comfort, but in two cases—ovarian carcinomas and lymphoma—it may well respond to treatment of the underlying condition.

Management

◆ Therapeutic paracentesis is often required and the immediate comfort produced is much appreciated by the patient. It has to be remembered that when the 'cushioning effect' of the ascites has been removed, the patient may experience pain in the enlarged liver and tumour masses. There is no means of predicting how often the procedure will need to be repeated. If it is frequent enough to be exhausting for the patient being taken back and forth to the hospital or palliative care unit, consideration should be given to a drain being left in, draining into an abdominal bag. Always it should be remembered that the frequent removal of so much albumin would eventually lead to further oedema secondary to hypoalbuminaemia, which does not respond to replacement albumin infusions.

- Spironolactone, 100–400 milligrams daily, is useful to slow down the reaccumulation of ascites, but at the cost of anorexia in most patients and gynaecomastia in males. Frusemide in mega doses (250–500 milligrams) is not recommended even in cardiac patients. The diuresis distresses the patient and there might develop electrolyte imbalance, hepatic encephalopathy, or pre-renal failure.

- Perito-venous shunts can be inserted, draining the fluid from the abdomen to the internal jugular vein. It is not recommended. Results are poor in malignant disease with an operative mortality of 15 per cent, and 30 per cent in liver disease. The benefit only lasts 3–4 weeks.

Bladder problems

Bladder problems are common and can usually be managed in the home. Urinary incontinence does not usually lead to a request for hospital admission whereas faecal incontinence often does.

Incontinence

1. Urinary tract infection (UTI) is worth treating if the patient does not have an indwelling catheter in which case it is inappropriate. The patient with such a catheter should have weekly bladder lavage with normal saline, a procedure many will do for themselves after instruction.

2. Retention with overflow, if not due to prostatic hypertrophy, usually suggests a spinal cord compression, which demands urgent attention. It can also be caused by opioids .

3. Incontinence resulting from structural changes secondary to tumour, surgery, or radiotherapy is not amenable to treatment. The patient will need urinary diversion or a suprapubic catheter.

4. Excessive sedation, from whatever cause, can lead to incontinence.

Urinary retention

This may be caused by the following, and treated accordingly:

- anticholinergic drugs, tricyclic antidepressants, and the opioids;

- neurological problems such as spinal cord compression, tumour infiltration, damage to the pre-sacral plexuses;

- faecal impaction is common, however much the patient may deny constipation;

- prostatic obstruction in these patients will call for catheterization.

Dysuria and strangury

1. Infection dealt with as suggested above.
2. Generalized bladder pain responds to regular prostaglandin inhibitors such as naproxen (500 milligrams twice daily) or diclofenac (50 milligrams three times a day). Occasionally opioids will be necessary.
3. Strangury is more difficult to relieve. Occasionally propantheline (15 milligrams three times a day) or hyoscine butylbromide (20–120 milligrams a day via a syringe driver) will help. As a last resort a nerve block may be tried.

Haematuria

Here we are referring to haematuria from an already diagnosed, and treated, cause.

1. Palliative radiotherapy may relieve haematuria arising in a transitional cell bladder carcinoma.
2. Ethamsylate (500 milligrams four times a day) is effective in reducing capillary bleeding within 3–4 days.

Bladder washouts

Normal saline is used for routine weekly lavage in the catheterized patient when there is debris or clots. When infection is present, chlorhexidine 1:5000 is preferable, or noxytiolin as a week's course.

The primary care team need have no hesitations about catheterizing patients at home and caring for them in this way.

Breathlessness

Dyspnoea affects between 40–60 per cent of patients at the end of life. It is very subjective, with people reporting that they feel breathless yet not appearing to be dyspnoeic to onlookers, and vice versa. Nevertheless, this emphasizes its importance in palliative care because it matters to the patient who is likely to be very apprehensive and frightened. Unlike pain it is not easy to manage.

Causes

◆ Cardiac conditions such as cardiac failure, pericardial effusion, cardio-myopathy
◆ Respiratory conditions such as infection, effusion, bronchial obstruction, chronic obstructive pulmonary disease (COPD), and troublesome cough, superior vena caval obstruction (SVCO)

- ◆ Haematological conditions such as anaemia, reticuloses
- ◆ Neuromuscular conditions such as motor neurone disease
- ◆ Anxiety state
- ◆ Elevation of the diaphragm as a result of hepatomegaly, ascites, colonic distension.

Management

1. Identify the cause(s) and treat appropriately. Of course, this is easier said than done. The cardiac state may be such that medication is no longer helping. The lymphoma may no longer be responding to chemotherapy, the motor neurone disease be so advanced that symptom relief is all that can be offered, and the offending hepatomegaly cannot be reduced in size. Nevertheless, the list shows that there are often things which can be done whether it is tapping a pleural effusion or ascites, relieving a persistent cough, or helping the anxious person.

2. Apart from the specific treatments there are general measures which can help. The community nurse and physiotherapist may advise on relaxation, positioning, and breathing exercises, in addition to looking at ways to modify activities to accommodate the limitations imposed by dyspnoea.

3. The opioids are undoubtedly the best drugs for tachypnoea. When used on a regular basis and in the lowest dose found to be effective they do not depress respiration. This action on tachypnoea is specific and not a side-benefit of respiratory depression. It is well to remember when prescribing them that renal function is more important than hepatic, and that the younger the patient the higher the dose which will be required.

4. Start with oral morphine 5 milligrams every 4 hours round the clock except in the elderly where the starting dose is 2.5 milligrams. If the patient is already on morphine as an analgesic the dose should be increased by 50 per cent. Only when the maintenance dose has been defined can the patient be transferred to a slow-release preparation. There has been recent interest in administration of nebulized morphine, but at present there is no strong evidence for its efficacy.

5. Anxiolytics are occasionally needed even for patients on opioids. For immediate effect use lorazepam 0.5–1 milligrams sublingually. Should a more sustained effect be needed use diazepam 2–5 milligrams each night.

6. Dyspnoeic panic attacks are best relieved with midazolam 2.5–5 milligrams subcutaneously as described in the chapter on emergencies.

7. Oxygen is only indicated for anoxia, not for breathlessness per se. This is contrary to what many lay people believe because they have seen it save lives in television dramas and documentaries. The family doctor may be faced by a demand that the patient is given oxygen in the home, and if that is not acceded to, they ask for admission. It is often helpful to spend time explaining that oxygen is like a drug—useful for a few conditions but contraindicated in others where it might even do harm.

Confusion

At one time or another in their terminal illness close to 40 per cent of people will suffer some confusion. This is probably higher than many doctors and nurses expect and it is certainly not something most patients and their relatives anticipate. Understandably, both see it as a feature of mental illness, something even more difficult to accept than the physical illness, and one with a stigma attached. It is no wonder that confusion so often leads to a request for the patient to be readmitted to hospital or hospice.

Experience shows that, perhaps surprisingly, many relatives appreciate being warned in advance that confusion may develop. This may also help them to see that it is not caused by the drugs the patient is on, something they always seem to assume.

Causes

See Table 2.1.

Management

Clearly many of these causes are reversible, in which case every effort should be made to correct the cause. In acute attacks the most likely causes are shown in Table 2.1 in bold type.

1. Review all medication, looking particularly at steroids and benzodiazepines. Changing to an alternative may relieve the confusion.

2. The opioids may be a causative factor when they are given as bolus injections. Either change to subcutaneous via a syringe driver or try switching to another opioid.

Table 2.1 Causes of confusion

Infection

Raised intracranial pressure
Primary brain tumour
Secondary brain tumour

Hypoxia

Drug-induced
Anticholinergic drugs
Benzodiazepines
CNS stimulants
H2 antagonists
Opioids
Phenothiazines
Steroids

Metabolic
Hypercalcaemia
Hyponatraemia
Uraemia (chronic or acute-on-chronic)
Hepatic failure
Hyper- or hypoglycaemia
Hypothyroidism

Psychotic reaction to illness

Anaemia
Iron deficiency
B_{12} deficiency

Constipation

Urinary retention

Depression
Withdrawal of alcohol or drug after long-term dependency

3. Consider a neuroleptic particularly if there are psychotic features such as hallucinations or delusions. In the younger patients the preferable one is haloperidol 1.5–5 milligrams once daily unless rapid sedation is needed when it may be given subcutaneously. Elderly patients often do better on thioridazine, 10–25 milligrams three times a day, but, if sedation is called for, methotrimeprazine 12.5–25 milligrams is an alternative.

4. Care should be taken when using the benzodiazepines. They can occasionally exacerbate the confusion and, of course, if midazolam is used, with its marked amnesogenic effect, the patient becomes even more upset by the amnesia. However, it is probably the best drug if absolute sedation and tranquillity is needed in the final days.

As important as any medical intervention is the environment. Each member of the family must be spoken to, told what is thought to be causing the confusion, reassured that it is not a feature of a psychotic episode, and advised how to speak to the patient and respond to his/her questions. So often relatives feel they must correct confused ideas and misunderstandings, only adding to the patient's distress and embarrassment. Above all else, they must be shown how to create an atmosphere of peace and safety, one familiar to the patient if possible.

Transferring to a hospital or palliative care should be the last resort. It will inevitably entail moving to strange surroundings, getting to know and trust new carers—all of which will very likely increase the confusion rather than relieve it.

Constipation

This affects close on 90 per cent of the terminally ill. It is usually not taken as seriously as it deserves to be by doctors, is often mishandled by nurses, and both parties see the other as responsible for it and blame them accordingly. Very often the only person who takes it seriously is the patient.

Common causes
Dietary
  Inadequate roughage
  'Invalid' foods
  Inadequate fluid intake

Drug induced

 Opioids

 Tricyclic antidepressants

Immobility

Management

In many patients all of the above factors can be indicted but few changes can be made. As the illness progresses patients will not happily change to a high fibre diet and taking more fluids may not be easy. Opioid rotation may be tried but most of the group are constipating. It is often possible to increase mobility but not sufficient to improve the bowel action. The situation is frustrating to all concerned, not least the patient who is often both more anxious than he admits and uncomfortable.

Sooner rather than later a laxative will be required. Before prescribing one the doctor or nurse must perform a rectal examination. This is obligatory, not optional. One of three things will be found on rectal examination.

1. *A rectum filled with hard faeces.* There is no logic in giving an oral peristaltic stimulant to evacuate rock-hard faecal masses from the rectum. In most cases it is also likely to be too painful and upsetting to the frail patient to remove them manually. The patient should be given an arachis oil retention enema at night, advised not to try to empty the bowel, and either two bisacodyl suppositories or a warm phosphate enema the following morning. The whole procedure usually needs to be repeated the following evening. The rationale of this regimen is that the hard masses are softened by the oil, then expelled by the bisacodyl which works higher up the bowel, and the rectum then refills with more hard masses which have been in the sigmoid colon. The procedure to be followed when the rectum is eventually found to be empty is described below.

2. *Empty ballooned rectum.* The examining finger can scarcely feel the wall of the rectum so ballooned is it, like a megacolon or Hirschprung's disease. It signifies a faecal mass at the recto-sigmoid junction, too high to be felt by the examining finger and too low to be felt on abdominal examination. Giving an osmotic laxative will make the situation worse, merely making the faecal mass larger and more difficult to expel. Enemata and suppositories which act in the rectum are also useless. If enemata are used then a high arachis oil enema may be followed by a high phosphate enema the following morning. The patient must be

given a peristaltic stimulant such as senna, bisacodyl, sodium picosulphate, or danthron to advance the mass into the lower rectum. When it is felt by the examining finger (daily rectal examinations are required at this stage) the regimen advised above must be followed.

3. *Empty collapsed rectum*. This suggests there is no faecal mass in the rectum or at the recto-sigmoid junction. Careful abdominal examination is needed to find if the descending colon is loaded. There are no indications here for any rectal treatment. An appropriate oral regimen is needed.

Laxative regimen

The maintenance regimen to be adopted depends on the following:

- the patient's ability to swallow tablets and liquids
- the underlying pathology, whether the bowel is at risk or if there could be subacute obstruction
- the fluid intake
- other medication being taken.

In palliative care there is no place for lubricant laxatives such as liquid paraffin. Osmotic laxatives are effective only if there is a good enough fluid intake, seldom the case in this group of patients. Peristaltic stimulants may produce colic and faecal incontinence in the elderly frail but are invaluable when combined with a faecal softener. In most cases, therefore, the most appropriate laxative will be senna or a combination of senna and docusate.

It cannot be stated strongly enough that it is not a kindness to the frail patient under palliative care to be given frequent suppositories or enemata. Bowel action and the care needed should be discussed regularly and scientifically by the doctor and nurse. Critical times when this is even more important are when opioid doses are increased, when prokinetic drugs are introduced, and when there is change in fluid intake or loss.

Cough

Even though so many of the mortal illnesses necessitating palliative care are respiratory conditions, cough is not a common problem. When it does occur, however, it can lead to a crisis in care at home because neither patient nor family get much rest or sleep. It can be assumed here that the cause of the cough is self-evident.

The critical question is whether or not the cough is productive.

Management of a productive cough

Such a cough is usually caused by infection (though not necessarily a bacterial one requiring antibiotics) or cardiac failure, often showing as paroxysmal nocturnal dyspnoea. The importance of the physiotherapist cannot be overstated here. It is worth getting one into the home to teach the patient and carers how to facilitate expectoration or drainage of the chest.

Antibiotics have a place in palliative care, particularly when infected sputum is tenacious, making expectoration difficult. In practice, it is satisfactory to give an appropriate broad-spectrum antibiotic.

Management of a dry, unproductive cough

Particularly with an underlying malignancy such a cough can be very disturbing, keeping the patient and family awake at night, distressing when he is eating, and physically exhausting. Carers soon feel helpless, fear that death might occur as a result of the coughing, and assume that care would be better in hospital or a palliative care unit.

1. Cough suppressants such as codeine linctus, methadone linctus, pholcodeine, and codeine are worth trying but seldom work in these cases. If the patient is already on an opioid for analgesia, the cough needs to be increased by 50 per cent for cough suppression, but even this may not be effective.

2. Humidification of the atmosphere often helps. Gas and electric fires tend to dry the atmosphere more than fuel fires. Best of all, if the patient can use one, is a nebulizer with saline in the chamber, used every 4 hours.

3. If it is thought that the cough is caused, or exacerbated, by oedema surrounding a bronchial tumour, it can be relieved with steroids—dexamethasone 2–4 milligrams each morning. Nebulized bupivacaine, using 2 millilitres of 0.25 per cent every 4 hours may be helpful. The patient must be advised to breathe slowly and normally, not attempting to take deep breaths, and not to take food or fluids for 30 minutes after the inhalation.

4. Even attention to the positioning of the patient can make a difference. Patients with COPD prefer to sit upright in bed or a chair while those with a bronchogenic carcinoma prefer to be less upright, using only two or three pillows. The patient with a small pleural effusion will ask to lie on the side of the effusion unless it is painful where the

paracentesis needle was inserted. Most coughing, dyspnoeic patients prefer their comfortable armchair to being nursed in bed.

Depression

Most authorities now feel that depression in this group of patients is commoner than used to be thought, that it is often missed, and even when recognized is often undertreated. It seems to be important enough to merit treatment in not less than 20 per cent of palliative care patients.

There are several reasons for this underdiagnosis, and undertreatment. Doctors and nurses feel that terminally ill patients have every right to feel depressed. It is a normal response just as sadness is, and the two are often regarded as synonymous. Many of the medications used in depression have unpleasant side-effects such as dry mouth, constipation, and drowsiness, which add to the patient's burden. To this must be added the 10-day lag before benefit is experienced and such patients do not have time on their side.

The cardinal symptoms of a depressive state are well known but in terminal illness there are some which feature so consistently that they can be used as diagnostic markers—low self-esteem, poor sleep pattern, suicidal ideation, and poor or no concentration. Anyone who feels that they do not deserve care, that doctors and nurses would be better employed looking after others, and who sleeps badly is suffering from a depressive state.

Management

1. The first responsibility of the doctor and nurse is to have a high level of diagnostic suspicion throughout the whole time they are providing palliative care. Depression can creep on insidiously and easily go undetected.

2. The second responsibility is to ensure that all suffering is as well palliated as is possible. It is well recognized that depression is commoner in those with inadequately relieved symptoms.

3. There is still no agreement about whether it is preferable to start the patient on a tricyclic drug or one of the newer selective serotonin reuptake inhibitors (SSRIs).

4. The first SSRI to be tried would be fluoxetine taken in the morning . It does have to be remembered, however, that fluoxetine can cause nausea, anxiety, and appetite suppression (none of which are pleasant for patients at that stage of life) and that its half-life is 7–14 days.

5. The tricyclics should be used in lower doses than would be used in the physically healthy. For example, amitriptyline would be given as 75–125 milligrams a day. Amitriptyline and doxepin are best for the agitated, depressed patient with insomnia. Clomipramine is an alternative tricyclic when obsessional and phobic anxiety symptoms are present.

6. It is important to be able to reassure relatives that, to many people's surprise, suicide is very rare in this group of patients. Such attempts are almost always associated with premorbid psychopathology and/or a long-recognized personality disorder showing itself in hysterical or manipulative behaviour.

Diarrhoea

True diarrhoea only occurs in 4 per cent of palliative cancer patients referred to specialist units. Spurious diarrhoea, however, is very common and is almost always caused by faecal impaction. On the other hand, diarrhoea is a major problem in many AIDS patients.

Causes

1. Spurious—due to faecal impaction. This is so common that it might be made a rule of palliative care that all diarrhoea is spurious until proved otherwise. The need for rectal examination has been stressed in the section on constipation. If there is doubt about the level of impaction a straight film of abdomen should be ordered or, after discussion with the radiologist, a gastrographin enema which will define colonic pathology and act as a laxative.

2. Infection, as at any time in life. In AIDS patients cryptosporidiosis will be the cause in one-third of cases, salmonella may be difficult to treat but cytomegalovirus colitis is treatable.

3. Inflammatory bowel disease will probably be known to the patient before the terminal illness.

4. Internal fistulae (ileocolic or colocolic) are relatively common in malignant disease. They should be suspected in any patient with bowel or bladder carcinoma, when diarrhoea develops suddenly, no loading is seen on straight films, no organisms are found, and there is no response to antidiarrhoea treatment.

5. Excessive laxatives, either prescribed by the doctor, or taken in greater doses than recommended, or when the patient takes over-the-counter preparations.

Management

◆ Uncontrollable diarrhoea, particularly when the patient is at home, is a disaster. It is deeply upsetting and embarrassing for the patient, to say nothing about the fatigue it produces. For most relatives it is the proverbial straw that broke the camel's back and hospital admission is requested, with good reason. Both doctor and nurse should never hesitate about agreeing to such an admission. In the same way they should never withhold treatment in the home. Energetic treatment is essential.

◆ Identify and treat the cause must be the first rule.

◆ Prescribe antidiarrhoeals such as loperamide 4 milligrams as required, remembering that it can be given p.r.n. (as occasion may require), but occasionally a patient needs 4 milligrams every 4 hours. Diphenoxylate 5 milligrams three times a day is less effective than loperamide and can cause dry mouth, drowsiness, and light-headedness. It should be avoided in the elderly because of its ability to produce confusional states.

◆ There is little place for traditional kaolin mixtures in these patients.

◆ Codeine phosphate 30–60 milligrams three times a day is an effective and inexpensive constipating agent but it produces loculation of the faeces and soon the patient can go from liquid motions to faecal 'golf balls'.

◆ If the 'diarrhoea' is in fact steatorrhoea secondary to pancreatic carcinoma or chronic pancreatitis, the drug of choice is pancreatic extract, taken with meals. This is a timely reminder that a careful history is essential when investigating diarrhoea because steatorrhoea is frightening to patients who suspect that the greasy stools adhering to the toilet contain cancer cells, but it is eminently treatable.

◆ Methylcellulose, in tablet or granular form, is valuable for patients with diverticular disease but unable to take high roughage diet.

◆ One of the most useful drugs to have been introduced into palliative care in recent years is octreotide, a somatostatin analogue. It is valuable for high fluid output diarrhoea. The family doctor who wants advice about it should phone the local palliative medicine consultant and not attempt to start it at home without such advice.

Dry mouth

Dry mouth (xerostomia) is a common problem in patients receiving palliative care. Perhaps it does not sound important enough to merit a section in this book but it is uncomfortable, can sometimes be painful if there is secondary stomatitis, makes swallowing and speaking difficult, and can lead to halitosis which further isolates the patient.

Causes

+ Most of the commonly used medications, especially those with anticholinergic side-effects, dry the mouth mucus membranes.
+ A dry, centrally heated atmosphere that is now such a feature of homes as well as institutions.
+ Mouth breathing, itself usually the result of the dried nasal membranes.
+ Oxygen therapy, by nasal prongs or face masks.

Management

+ Proprietary preparations, usually sprays, are now available and effective for short periods.
+ Humidification of the atmosphere helps, whether achieved with a commercial unit or with a simple fine spray such as those used on household plants.
+ Sucking crushed ice helps the bedbound patient, particularly if it is flavoured.
+ Sweets have a temporary benefit but the flavour soon becomes nauseating.
+ The mouth must be checked at every visit of doctor or nurse to see that infection, and in particular candidiasis, has not developed.

Dysphagia

This is a more common problem than might be expected, with 12–23 per cent of patients reporting it, according to different surveys.

Causes

+ Pharyngeal obstruction secondary to intrinsic pressure from tumour mass, oedema, infection, or external pressure from tumour or nodes.
+ Oesophageal candidiasis (making swallowing painful rather than difficult), with symptoms resembling hiatus hernia or acid reflux.

* Oesophageal obstruction, intrinsically from tumour, stenosis, blocked oesophageal stent or externally from enlarged mediastinal nodes or (less commonly pleural effusion).
* Neuromuscular dysfunction, as in motor neurone disease and some of the rarer myopathies.

Management

It will be noticed that several of the causes listed will have been dealt with as part of the primary treatment, while others develop later in the course of the illness, even under palliative care in the home. A stent can easily block; candidiasis develops rapidly in the frail and immuno-compromised; nodes can be involved with tumour and soon cause extrinsic pressure. The doctor and nurse need to be on constant alert for such events in their patients with these underlying conditions.

* Oesophagitis as a result of candida usually occurs because the patient has not been instructed to swallow the nystatin suspension after swilling it round the mouth. If this has not been the case a different antifungal should be prescribed.

* When due to radiation, the pain of oesophagitis will usually subside spontaneously, but if not, an antacid containing a surface anaesthetic, such as mucaine, will be adequate or an opioid combined with ompeprazole.

* When an oesophageal stent (Celestin or Atkinson) blocks there is usually no alternative to referring the patient back to hospital to have it cleaned out endoscopically and then the patient can return home. Far better is to prevent the blockage by giving the correct advice on diet and lubrication when eating!

The patient should be instructed to drink some water before every mouthful of food. Plain water is adequate but carbonated water may feel more reassuring to the patient. The diet must be 'anything you would normally eat with a spoon' and contain no chunks of meat, no doughy bread (even as sandwiches), and no dry food.

Other simple advice is to eat one course at a meal, to eat as much ice cream or sorbet as possible, and to stand for about 10 minutes after each meal, rather than lounging in a chair, to encourage better gastric emptying.

* Laser therapy is being offered increasingly to widen the lumen before suggesting a stent. The patient needs to be advised that the dysphagia will be worse for about 24 hours after the procedure, but will then improve considerably.

◆ Mediastinal adenopathy, developing in someone too frail to return to hospital, not keen to do so, or who has already had maximal irradiation there, may respond to dexamethasone, 8 milligrams each morning until a response is seen, then reduced slowly to a maintenance dose of 2 milligrams daily.

Faecal incontinence

It is a well-observed fact that relatives are often willing to care for a loved one with urinary incontinence but not with faecal incontinence, even when nurses are attending, the facilities in the house are good, and there is a special laundry service. More than 20 per cent of people admitted to specialist palliative care units are faecally incontinent.

Causes

1. In the elderly lax anal sphincters are often to blame.
2. In most palliative care patients the cause is spurious diarrhoea secondary to faecal impaction.
3. Both young and old occasionally take excessive prescribed laxatives, or over-the-counter preparations containing peristaltic stimulants or liquid paraffin or phenolphthalein.
4. The incontinence may not be faecal but an offensive mucous discharge from an anal carcinoma.

Management

◆ A careful rectal examination is mandatory (see section on constipation). No surgical treatment will improve the lax sphincter but an agent to firm up the stool will help—loperamide, methylcellulose, or codeine phosphate.

◆ Surgical treatment, in the form of a defunctioning colostomy, does have a place in the patient suffering an anal discharge from a rectal or anal carcinoma.

If the surgeon does not feel that a colostomy is appropriate then there remain the options of laser therapy or irradiation, particularly if the tumour is fungating or bleeding.

◆ Anal discharge and discomfort can be eased with rectal steroids (suppositories or retention enemata) twice daily.

Obvious as it sounds, the patient can be prescribed incontinence pads. Many are unaware that they can be prescribed and improvise in some way.

◆ Paraplegic patients present a different problem. It is often better to make them constipated and perform manual evacuation twice weekly rather than risk incontinence after they have had laxatives.

Halitosis

This is a common problem but rarely reported by patients, who may either be unaware of it or think doctors are not interested in it because they never enquire about it. Occasionally a relative will mention this as a reason they do not bring grandchildren to see the patient or why they themselves find visiting embarrassing.

Causes

1. Diseases of the mouth, gums, teeth, and/or poor oral hygiene, particularly in mouth breathers and those with xerostomia.

2. Diseases of the upper respiratory tract, particularly the sinuses.

3. Diseases of the lower respiratory tract particularly bronchiectasis, lung abscess, and secondary infection in a necrotizing cavity or lung tumour.

4. Diseases of the stomach, particularly when there is delayed gastric emptying ('cesspool halitosis') or linitis plastica.

5. Metabolic disorders such as diabetic ketoacidosis, uraemia, and hepatic failure with obstructive jaundice.

6. In those still managing a 'normal' diet one thinks of curried food, garlic, onions, etc.

Management

◆ Clearly some of the commonest causes can be corrected or given additional attention. e.g. oral hygiene.

◆ Prokinetic drugs (metoclopramide, cisapride) should be given for gastric stasis.

◆ Metronidazole 200 milligrams three times a day is highly effective for odours arising in the lower respiratory tract even when sensitivities have not been possible.

◆ Very often one has to return to sucking peppermint sweets!

Hiccup

Trivial as this symptom may sound, it can prevent a patient eating or enjoying a meal, can provoke vomiting, will upset relatives who feel helpless to do anything, and can persist for days, leaving the patient exhausted. For some reason it is commoner in women than in men and, in spite of the causes listed below, is usually psychogenic.

Causes

1. Irritation of the phrenic nerve anywhere in its course but particularly near the hilum where it can be affected by tumour.
2. Irritation of the diaphragm by infection or tumour.
3. Uraemia.
4. Dyspepsia, especially with hiatus hernia, gastric stasis, and aerophagy (probably the commonest cause in the terminally ill).
5. Elevation of the diaphragm as a result of ascites or massive hepatomegaly.
6. Raised intracranial pressure or cerebrovascular disease (the commonest physical cause in the elderly and those with non-fatal illness).

Management

♦ When possible identify and treat the cause. Except for uraemia and infection this is seldom possible.
♦ All of the following medications have been tried and found to be effective at some time or another:
  ♦ a defoaming antiflatulent before and after each meal;
  ♦ chlorpromazine 10–25 milligrams orally three times a day;
  ♦ prokinetic drugs when the cause is gastric distension, e.g. metoclopramide 10 milligrams three times a day;
  ♦ baclofen 5 milligrams twice daily, but doses as high as 20 milligrams three times a day have been used.

Hypercalcaemia

Estimates vary but this probably occurs in 5–10 per cent of cancer patients, predominantly but not exclusively in those with squamous cell disease, whether affecting bronchus, cervix, oesophagus, or any other site. It is often, but by no means always, associated with known bone metastases. It is a very uncommon condition in other terminal illnesses.

It should be suspected in any patient with a squamous carcinoma who develops:

+ sudden onset of confusion or vagueness;
+ extreme thirst and polyuria;
+ rapidly worsening fatigue, listlessness, apathy, and generalized flaccidity.

These might be regarded as the features of malignancy, but in hypercalcaemia they develop rapidly, often over a few days. They might also be thought to be the features of a depressive state, but missing are low self-esteem and poor sleep pattern. Doctors and nurses providing palliative care in the home must have a high level of diagnostic suspicion to detect hypercalaemia and be ready to take blood for calcium and albumin estimations to confirm their suspicions.

Management

Whether or not to treat hypercalcaemia, to have the patient admitted for treatment, or to try to provide it in the home are important and difficult ethical decisions. Improvement with bisphosphonates and intravenous rehydration is seen within 2 days, after which the patient usually returns home. Whether this is appropriate treatment depends on how ill the person is, what prognosis he was thought to have before the onset of the hypercalcaemia, how well the family members are coping, what journey is involved in getting the patient to hospital, and what other problems are currently being palliated. The list is a long one but this ethical challenge cannot be avoided.

If the symptoms have developed relatively slowly improvement will also be less rapid and dramatic. If the hypercalcaemia is almost a coincidental event in a patient with many other much more distressing and difficult-to-palliate symptoms, transfer to hospital may be a burden rather than a blessing. On the other hand, energetic treatment for the underlying pathology (for example, radiotherapy for the carcinoma) is well worth-while for the person thought to have a long enough prognosis.

The only effective treatment is intravenous saline rehydration and intravenous bisphosphonates. Biochemical improvement is seen within a few days and visible improvement in the patient after that. When the patient comes home it must be remembered that serum calcium levels will rise again between day 21 and day 28 when the whole procedure may have to be repeated.

It is now recognized that little benefit follows the use in the home of high-dose steroids and withholding milk confers no benefit whatsoever.

Insomnia

Approximately 70 per cent of our patients report insomnia. Presumably the same proportion of caring relatives and friends also experience it, for it is difficult to sleep when the person you are caring for is wide awake and possibly distressed because of it. It takes only a few wakeful, exhausting nights to make relatives suggest admission for the patient. Little do most people appreciate how difficult it is to sleep in a noisy hospital ward!

Causes

- Any physical distress, whether it is pain, pressure sores, pruritus, cough, urinary frequency, or anything else.

- Depression. Classically there is early morning wakening but often this is not as distressing for the patient as the shallowness of the sleep.

- Hallucinations and nightmares, very occasionally features of a psychotic illness but in palliative care patients much more likely to be due to medication (H2 antagonists, benzodiazepines, and steroids taken late in the day).

- Cerebral pathology, particularly primary brain tumours, with reversal of sleep rhythms, turning day into night and vice versa.

- Anxiety and fears, possibly mentioned to the doctor or nurse, but often unventilated in case they sound trivial.

- Night sweats, usually due to advanced carcinoma with liver secondaries, or one of the reticuloses, or a chronic infection such as tuberculosis, AIDS and its opportunistic infections.

- Drug withdrawal, particularly of the benzodiazepines, barbiturates, and opioids, when the patient has been taking them for some considerable time.

Management

It cannot be stated strongly enough that every possible physical cause must be looked for and treated appropriately. Pain that can be borne silently during the day can become unbearable at night. It a useful rule that pain experienced both during the day and at night (though not necessarily reported during the day) is organic in nature. Pain experienced only at night is almost always psychogenic. This does not make it any less unpleasant or less worthy of treatment but it points to the need to explore fears and depression rather than prescribing opioids.

It has also to be remembered that it may be 'trivial' things that keep a person awake—sweating copiously, pruritus, creases in bedclothes, and so forth.

There are patients who will themselves not to sleep, having been reassured by their well-intentioned doctors that dying is just as peaceful as dropping off to sleep.

Poor sleep may be the first and, for a time, the only feature of a developing depressive state. When no other cause can be identified, the doctor and nurse should make a note to keep checking for features of developing depression.

Two commonly prescribed drugs can lead to disturbed sleep. Diuretics taken late in the day can disturb because of the need to pass water. Dexamethasone taken in the late afternoon or evening is guaranteed to stimulate the patient and probably induce agitation and nightmares.

The environment where the patient is being cared for needs attention. The doctor and nurse will wish to check that there is no unnecessary background noise, no sound from televisions in nearby rooms, no traffic noise. It might be found useful to have some of the patient's favourite music playing in the background. Whether or not the patient is better nursed in bed or in an armchair has to be discussed. Most with pulmonary conditions prefer to be propped up in a chair. If they have a pleural effusion they choose to lie on the affected side.

Only when everything else has been looked into do you turn to sedatives. Benzodiazepines are preferable, in short half-life formulations. If a person has been a long-term benzodiazepine taker, there is nothing to be gained by trying to wean them off them and substitute with something else at this stage in life.

If there is any suggestion that the patient has a depressive illness then the best drug is a tricyclic antidepressant with sedative properties.

Intestinal obstruction

It is assumed that the diagnosis is known beyond any doubt. What follows are guidelines for the management of the patient who subsequently develops obstruction. The basic question for the family doctor and nurse are whether or not care can and should be given in the home. Although the hospital management is not their responsibility, they nevertheless must know it and be able both to advise the patient and carers. It can be summarized as follows.

Gastric outlet obstruction

No sooner has the patient swallowed a mouthful of food or fluid than it is vomited up and the patient feels comfortable and ready to tackle another mouthful. There is no nausea, usually no pain, and nothing to find on examination.

The patient must be admitted to hospital. If there is no colic, a trial of steroids and metoclopramide may be effective. If this fails, then nasogastric suction will be needed, and possibly intravenous fluids. Attempts will be made to identify the cause. If an operation is done it will probably be the creation of a palliative gastro-enterostomy.

Small bowel obstruction

Whether or not this patient is admitted to hospital depends on:

1. whether it is thought there is a single site of obstruction (in which case surgical relief might be called for) or multiple sites (when surgical intervention is not going to help);

2. whether it is a total or a subtotal obstruction (is flatus being passed?). If total, admission will be needed. If subtotal, conservative management can be given at home;

3. how dehydrated the patient is. If seriously so, then admission is needed unless the doctor and nurse are happy to give subcutaneous fluids in the house, a perfectly easy and acceptable thing to do.

It is important to remember that pain can be controlled as easily at home as in a hospital; that it is not mandatory to give 'drip and suction', and that very adequate volumes of fluids can be taken by mouth and absorbed when the site of the obstruction is low in the bowel. Close on 1 litre of saline per day can be given subcutaneously in the home by using a butterfly needle.

Large bowel obstruction

The clinical features are pathognomonic. The obstruction develops slowly, flatus is passed until the late stages, nausea is seldom a problem, and vomiting may be delayed for days before the classical faecal-smelling vomitus comes up. Colic develops slowly but may be severe. The flanks are distended with tympany on percussion.

In palliative care these patients can usually be cared for at home without 'drip and suction', their bowels kept moving by the use of docusate, their pain controlled with hyoscine butylbromide 20 milligrams every 4 hours or 120 milligrams a day via a syringe driver with the addition of diamorphine. Fluids may be taken by mouth in the form of short drinks, sucking iced lollipops, crushed ice cubes, and fruit juices. If vomiting is a problem then cyclizine or haloperidol may be effective in the syringe driver.

This decision making is difficult. Most doctors and nurses have been brought up to think that the only treatment is 'drip and suction', which is synonymous with hospital admission. The possibility of managing a subcutaneous infusion in the home has often never been considered. It is also well recognized that when such a patient goes to hospital little consideration or discretion will be employed, and within minutes not only will drip and suction be instituted but arrangements made for daily electrolyte profiles, radiology, scanning, and even review by the surgeons in case laparotomy is called for. This is a daunting prospect for the patient known to have advanced malignancy and eager just to be as comfortable as possible with the least 'interference'.

Lymphangitis carcinomatosis

This may not be common but it is terrifying for the patients, most of whom have breast carcinoma. Dyspnoea worsens inexorably until it is disabling at rest. Cough is not a regular feature but when it occurs it is dry and totally non-productive. The only signs are the fine crepitations to be heard throughout the chest, much finer than those of cardiac failure. Chest films may show characteristic change but are more usually of no help whatsoever. Essentially this is a diagnosis based on suspicion when caring for a person at risk.

Management

If there is any possibility that this is a chemotherapy-sensitive carcinoma the case should be discussed with the oncologist. Very likely the patient has had all the chemotherapy possible but it is worth exploring.

Steroids are the only drugs found to have an appreciably beneficial effect. The family doctor should not hesitate to start them, not waiting to discuss this with specialists. Preferable is dexamethasone 4 milligrams each morning (divided into equal doses early morning and midday if so desired) and maintained at that dose permanently. As in other causes of dyspnoea in palliative care, opioids reduce the tachypnoea but not as satisfactorily as in pulmonary metastases.

In the final stages, so severe is the dyspnoea and so frightening, the doctor is justified in prescribing a tranquillizer along with the opioid, midazolam being the best when a syringe driver is in use.

Lymphoedema

See Chapter 10.

Nausea and vomiting

Two observations are worth making at the outset. Nausea distresses patients even more than vomiting and it often proves more difficult to treat than any other symptom in the palliative care patient. That is not to imply that vomiting is unimportant but, provided the patient does not experience nausea as well as vomiting and can proceed to take some food or fluid after a vomit, he is not unduly distressed by it. Persistent nausea produces a worse sense of helplessness than almost anything else.

Causes

In approximately 50 per cent of cases no definite cause can be found and treatment has to be empirical. It is safe in most cases to assume that several things are producing the nausea:

1. *Metabolic*: hyper- or hyponatraemia, hypercalcaemia, uraemia.

2. *Drug-induced*: any and every drug employed in medicine can produce nausea and vomiting. Traditionally the opioids are blamed in palliative care patients but this is unfair—they only induce nausea in the first few days of use, when the dose has to be increased rapidly, and when the starting dose was excessively high. With these exceptions the opioids should not be blamed. This is of great importance because, as every doctor and nurse learns, we still encounter opiophobia and patients and relatives grasp at any reason for discontinuing these drugs. Whenever drugs are thought to be implicated, the doctor and nurse should check on renal function and urine output, nausea often being related to poor clearance and elimination.

3. *Intestinal obstruction*: this has been dealt with in this chapter.

4. *Raised intracranial pressure*: this is suggested when vomiting (usually without nausea) occurs, particularly in the morning accompanied by

headache, fits, and focal neurological features. The first hint of it may be the vomiting. Papilloedema may be seen on examination.

5. *Chronic constipation*: although the authors would not go so far as to name this as the principal cause of nausea and vomiting, it is certainly a major contributory factor.

6. *Anxiety and fear*: unless one thing stands out as the cause then it is always worth exploring the patient's anxieties and fears, calm and philosophic as they may appear.

7. *Cardiac failure*: congestion can cause nausea, but it will always be accompanied by other features such as dyspnoea, basal crepitations, raised jugular venous pressure (JVP), etc.

Management

See Table 2.2.

1. As always, try to identify a cause before rushing in to prescribe an antiemetic.

2. The best non-specific antiemetic (as well as being the best for drug-induced nausea) is haloperidol 0.5–1.5 milligrams nightly (bearing in mind its long half-life). Rarely is it necessary to resort to doses higher than 5 milligrams over 24 hours.

3. The preferable one for obstruction, as part of the regimen outlined, is cyclizine 50 milligrams three times a day preferably subcutaneously, or via a syringe-driver (remembering that a dense white precipitate will be formed which is safe but which will block small needles).

4. For gastric outlet obstruction a prokinetic agent may be tried, such as metoclopramide, domperidone, or cisapride, after checking with the oncologist that no further chemotherapy is feasible. It is worth remembering that the traditional dose of metoclopramide 10 milligrams three times a day will be inadequate and should be replaced by 20 or 30 milligrams three times a day, although doses as high as 120 milligrams in 24 hours are now sometimes used in palliative care, the preferable route being subcutaneous by syringe driver.

What does the doctor or nurse do when everything has failed, as is not infrequent?

♦ Try again to identify the cause.

♦ Rationalize all medication to get it to the absolute minimum (remembering that in palliative care patients the average number of separate drugs they are on is 7.5).

Table 2.2 Antiemetics

Cause of nausea/ vomiting	Suggested drug	BNF Ref.	Preparations/ Comment
Metabolic	Haloperidol	4.2.1	Tabs 1.5 mg, 5 mg, 10 mg
Uraemia	PO 1.5 mg nocte		Liq. 2 mg/ml
Hypercalcaemia	SC 1.5–5 mg once daily		Inj. 5 mg/ml and 10 mg/ml
Drugs	Metoclopramide	4.6	Tabs 10 mg or 15 mg SR, 30 mg SR
	PO/SC 10–20 mg t.d.s. SC 30–100 mg/24 h		Sol. 5 mg/5 ml Inj. 10 mg/2 ml
Gastric stasis	Metoclopramide	4.6	Tabs 10 mg or 15 mg SR, 30 mg SR
	PO/SC 10–20 mg t.d.s. SC 30–100 mg/24 h		Sol. 5 mg/5 ml Inj. 10 mg/2 ml
	Dexamethasone 6 mg daily to see if response	6.3.2	
	Cisapride PO 10 mg tablets	1.3	Tabs 10 mg
Gastric irritation	Metoclopramide PO/SC 10–20 mg t.d.s. SC 30–100 mg/24 h	4.6	Asilone suspension Lansoprazole 30 mg od Omeprazole 20 mg od
Subacute bowel obstruction—	Metoclopramide SC 10–20 mg t.d.s.	4.6	Phosphate enema to empty lower colon Faecal softener, e.g. Docusate 100 mg t.d.s.
without colic	SC 30–100 mg/24 h via driver		
	Dexamethasone (add) SC 8–12 mg pre 6 p.m.	6.3.2	Beware stimulant laxatives
Subacute bowel obstruction— with colic	Cyclizine SC 100–150 mg/24 h Then add	4.6	Inj. 50 mg/ml
	Haloperidol SC 2.5–5 mg/24 h	4.2.1	
	Or substitute Methotrimeprazine SC 6.25–25 mg single dose or add 25–50 mg SC/24 h	4.2.1	6.25 mg–25 mg may be given by single SC injection

Table 2.2 (cont.)

Cause of nausea/ vomiting	Suggested drug	BNF Ref.	Preparations/ Comment
	Hyoscine butylbromide 60–120 mg/24 h for colic		Inj. 20 mg/ml
	Also consider trial of Dexamethasone 8–2 mg/24 h SC pre 6 p.m		Avoid stimulant laxatives
	Octreotide 300–600 μg/24 h Seek specialist advice		Avoid metoclopramide
Raised intracranial pressure	Dexamethasone PO/SC 8–16 mg SC p re 6 p.m. With	6.3.2	Single dose injection before 6 p.m.
	Cyclizine 50 mg t.d.s. or SD 150 mg SC/24 h	4.6	
Motion	Prochlorperazine PO 5 mg t.d.s. PR 25 mg bd IM 12.5 mg	4.6	Not for SC use Tabs 5 mg Supp. 25 mg Inj. 12.5 mg
Broad-spectrum antiemetics	Methotrimeprazine	4.2	Consider ondansetron IV or IM 8 mg PO 8 mg bd SC 8–16 mg/24 h Rectal

PO, by mouth; SC, subcutaneously; SR, slow release; SD, Syringe Driver; PR, per rectum; IM, intramuscularly; IV, intravenously.

Discuss it with the local palliative medicine consultant who may visit if requested to do so, or give advice or even suggest a few days in the palliative care unit where, surprisingly, the problem may resolve without ever finding the cause.

♦ Try adding another antiemetic of a different pharmaceutical family and observing over 3–4 days.

♦ Stopping all anti-emetics and, empirically, giving dexamethasone 4 milligrams each morning for 5 days then reducing to a maintenance dose of 2 milligrams daily.

LIVERPOOL JOHN MOORES UNIVERSITY
LEARNING & INFORMATION SERVICES

Night sweats

These are commoner than often realized, are worrying to patients who suspect they have infectious diseases as well as their malignancy, and greatly increase the work of the relatives and friends. Often the patient has to be changed frequently at night and soon the skin suffers and breaks down.

Causes

1. Hepatic metastases from any primary. The more enzymes secreted the worse the sweating. It is, of course, a recognized feature of the reticuloses.
2. Infection, whether primary, such as tuberculosis, or opportunistic, as in AIDS and the immuno-compromised cancer patient.
3. Sarcoidosis.

Management

Apart from trying to identify a cause, all treatment relates to hepatic activity.

◆ When the patient is so ill that death is considered imminent, all efforts are put into nursing, cooling, the use of fans, talc powder, appropriate bed linen, etc. Drugs have no place.

◆ When the liver enzymes are rising rapidly, yet the patient is remarkably well in spite of the extent of the underlying malignancy and is thought to have several months or weeks prognosis, then try H2 antagonists such as cimetidine or ranitidine in the usual doses. The response is usually excellent and the drugs can often be withdrawn, albeit temporarily.

◆ When the patient is frail, the enzymes are rising rapidly but the prognosis is only a few weeks give dexamethasone 4 milligrams each morning, reducing to 2 milligrams after a week or two if the patient is still alive.

◆ A trial of a non-steroidal anti-inflammatory drug (NSAID) may be effective, e.g. naproxen 500 milligrams twice a day.

Oedema

We shall look at this from an anatomical point of view.

◆ *Bilateral upper limb oedema* is superior vena caval obstruction until proved otherwise. Check for distension of collateral veins on the thoracic and upper abdominal wall, peri-orbital oedema, marked elevation of JVP, and very distressing dyspnoea. The management is dealt with on p. 85.

◆ *Unilateral upper limb oedema* is almost always lymphoedema (see p. 127). In patients who do not have the usual precursors of lymphoedema (breast carcinoma, radiotherapy, and surgery to the axilla), the possibility of axillary vein thrombosis has to be considered.

◆ *Unilateral lower limb oedema* may be caused by a deep vein thrombosis (DVT), venous obstruction at the level of the internal iliac veins, or lymphoedema, both secondary to local tumour or nodal involvement.

Management

Whether or not to treat DVT with anticoagulants is a difficult ethical decision. The doctor, in discussion with the nurse, will take into account the advanced nature of the underlying disease, the probable prognosis, the attitude of the patient to hospital admission, the ease or otherwise of monitoring an anticoagulant regimen at home on discharge against the dangers of emboli and infarction, and the logistics of home care.

If a community hospital is available then admission might be useful for a few days while anticoagulant control is established.

The issue of anticoagulation is not the only one. If venous obstruction is caused by radiosensitive tumour the patient might be made much more comfortable with a single fraction of radiotherapy. Clearly discussion with the oncologist is called for. Either the oncologist or the local palliative medicine consultant might recommend high-dose steroids to reduce tumour bulk, dexamethasone 8 milligrams each morning, reduced by 2 milligrams every 2 days.

◆ *Bilateral lower limb oedema* is caused by:

● cardiac failure, with all its classical features;

● pelvic obstruction from tumour and/or nodes which, if not already done, can be demonstrated on ultrasound scan (USS), computerized tomography (CT), or magnetic resonance imaging (MRI);

● hypoalbuminaemia from liver failure or repeated paracentesis abdominis.

Management

The cardiac failure is treated in the usual way but in palliative care patients is usually an end event and the relatives should be advised accordingly.

The pelvic obstruction calls for oncologist advice about irradiation and/or steroids. Diuretics are generally unhelpful.

The hypoalbuminaemia is a terminal event. Experiences show that albumin infusions at this late stage do not help to change the course of events or the patient's comfort. The only helpful measures, nursing ones, are elevation of the feet and legs, remembering that the oedema may simply move higher and affect thighs, external genitalia in the male, and buttocks, with the real possibility of the skin breaking down.

Pericardial effusion

This is rare. A family doctor may go through a lifetime of practice and never see a case. It is extremely distressing for the patient and palliative treatment is possible and helpful.

Causes

- ◆ Myocardial infarction
- ◆ Pericarditis (pyogenic, viral, and tuberculous)
- ◆ Malignancy, spreading from local tumours or nodes
- ◆ Metastatic from a distant malignancy.

The patient is exceedingly dyspnoeic, has muffled heart sounds, cardiac tamponade, and cardiac failure. Unless the patient is expected to die within hours or days, hospital admission to a cardiothoracic unit should be arranged for urgent paracentesis (either by aspiration or the creation of a pericardial window through the diaphragm).

If it is decided to keep the patient at home, the seriousness of the condition must be explained to relatives and the patient kept comfortable and probably heavily sedated with opioids and midazolam.

Pleural effusion

Pleural effusion is so common in palliative care patients and the benefits of paracentesis and/or pleurodesis so great that it is worth keeping this complication in mind when offering palliative care in the home.

Pleural effusion carries a poor prognosis for all malignant disease patients except women with breast carcinoma, where they may have it up to 18 months before death.

Unless the patient is thought to be in the final days of life, hospital admission for paracentesis is worthwhile to relieve dyspnoea.

If the effusion recurs within weeks, the paracentesis should be repeated and a pleurodesis attempted. Different units use different agents but those in commonest use are talc powder, tetracycline and, less often, bleomycin. It should be remembered that when the patient returns home they may be febrile, feel 'flu-like' and exhausted for a few days.

If the effusion is secondary to mesothelioma, paracentesis should only be done after much consideration. Tumour seedlings will grow in the needle tract, producing exquisitely painful nodules.

Pruritus

Causes

- ◆ Obstructive jaundice
- ◆ Hodgkin's lymphoma
- ◆ Myeloma
- ◆ Carcinoid syndrome
- ◆ Uraemia
- ◆ Opioids

Management

- ◆ Nursing input is essential to keep the skin cool and dry, and to guard against infection in scratch marks.
- ◆ Biliary stenting is the most effective measure for obstruction. Some jaundice may persist but all pruritus will go.
- ◆ If stenting is not feasible, cholestyramine should be tried, provided the patient can tolerate the taste. (It must be remembered that this drug will worsen any steatorrhoea.)
- ◆ Both H1 receptor blockers and phenothiazines occasionally relieve pruritus if the patient cannot tolerate cholestyramine but the sedative effects may not be acceptable.
- ◆ H2 receptor blockers have been shown to help.
- ◆ For night sedation, trimeprazine tartrate 10 milligrams is ideal.

- Topical steroids occasionally work but just as effective is dabbing the skin with a solution of sodium bicarbonate (one tablespoon in a cup of warm water) and allowing it to dry on the skin.
- Rifampicin is effective in primary biliary cirrhosis but not in any other pruritic condition.

Sore mouth

Causes

- Oral candidiasis, so common in advanced malignancy but less so in advanced cardiac, respiratory, and neurological disorders.
- Aphthous ulcers, less common than candidiasis but distressingly painful.
- Post chemotherapy/radiotherapy stomatitis.

Management

- Candidiasis usually responds to oral nystastin suspension provided dentures are taken out beforehand, the suspension is swilled around the mouth and then swallowed (to prevent oesophagitis), dentures are thoroughly cleaned, and the regimen is continued indefinitely. Only when this carefully monitored regimen fails should nystatin be changed to ketoconazole 200 milligrams daily or, more effective but much more costly, fluconazole 50 milligrams daily for 5 days.
- For aphthous ulcers the following are all effective:
  - tetracycline suspension mouthwash 10 millilitres rinse for 2 minutes before swallowing, repeated every 6 hours;
  - hydrocortisone pellets 2.5 milligrams sucked as close to the ulcer as possible four times a day;
  - Aschurt's solution (betamethasone solution) 5–10 millilitres every 4 hours (made up specially by the pharmacist);
  - herpetic ulcers (in AIDS) respond to acyclovir orally 200 milligrams every 4 hours for 5 days.
- Post-chemotherapy stomatitis clears spontaneously but comfort can be achieved with benzydamine mouthwash. Lignocaine gel is effective but must be used with care because of the danger of aspiration due to the anaesthesia.

Xerostomia produces no symptoms other than a dry mouth, making speech difficult. It does, however, lead to infections and ulceration. It is caused by mouth breathing, inadequate fluids, drugs with anticholinergic effects, and poor oral hygiene, all common problems in patients at home. It is surprisingly difficult to help but it is worth trying the following:

- sucking thin slices of chilled tinned (not fresh) pineapple;
- sugarless chewing gum or hydrophilic chewing gum;
- sucking crushed flavoured ice cubes or effervescent vitamin C tablets;
- artificial saliva.

It is worth remembering that when a patient has a dry and/or a sore mouth from whatever cause they prefer cold fluids to warm ones, semi-solids to solids. Even if they have not been fond of them when well, they will very likely appreciate ice creams and sorbets.

Superior vena caval obstruction (SVCO)

This will only be seen once or twice in the professional lifetime of a family doctor but it is so unpleasant and threatening for the patient and the treatment so successful, it is worth mentioning here.

It is caused by anything obstructing the superior vena cava as it approaches the right atrium, whether local tumour or nodes affected by carcinoma or one of the reticuloses. The patient reports increasing dyspnoea, rapidly curtailing all daily activities. Collateral veins course across the anterior chest wall and upper abdominal wall. Pads of oedema appear beneath the eyes, the face becomes bloated, and the arms swell up giving a grotesque appearance to the patient. The JVP is elevated.

Management

The urgent advice of a radiotherapist should be sought. Time should not be wasted having the patient admitted to a general ward. It might still be possible to irradiate the central chest or to give chemotherapy for a lymphoma if this symptom is a presenting feature.

Whether or not the patient is to have radiotherapy the doctor can and should give intramuscular dexamethasone 16 milligrams on day 1, reducing by 4 milligrams daily until it is discontinued by which time the SVCO will have improved.

Weakness and lethargy

It might be thought that these are inevitable features of all major illnesses, whatever the pathology, and would be accepted as such by patients and relatives. This is not so. Most patients seem unprepared for them even when they know about their malignancy, cardiac insufficiency, renal failure, or whatever else they have. They are often more upset by the weakness and the dependency it creates than by all the other features of the illness.

Likewise, relatives will plead for something to restore some energy even when they too know how serious the illness is. Unless this issue is addressed they will soon be asking for hospital admission, blood transfusion, dietary manipulation, total parenteral nutrition, or tonics.

Causes

Rather than simply saying weakness is inevitable it might help to look at some treatable causes.

* Anaemia.

* Excessive sedation: those without great experience in prescribing opioids often use doses that are higher than needed for analgesia and are sedative.

* Metabolic: uraemia, hypercalcaemia, hypo- and hypernatraemia.

* Adrenal failure due to malignant metastases in the adrenal or the patient's failure to take prescribed hydrocortisone after hypophysectomy, adrenalectomy, or aminoglutethamide (unusual as these are now).

* Depression: psychomotor retardation can easily be mistaken for generalized weakness and lethargy.

* Low grade infection, particularly in the typically immuno-compromised palliative care patient. This raises the ethical consideration as to how energetic the doctor should be in searching for the infection in such a patient.

* Boredom: it is a paradox that good palliative care may keep patients alive longer than expected (though it does not set out to extend life) but they are never energetic again, are readily exhausted, and soon become bored. This is one of the indications for Day Care, whether in the local Day Hospice or a similar facility operated by a charity or NHS trust. Palliative care patients, like all of us throughout life, want to be needed and valued, rather than a burden on loved ones and society. The Day Care facility responds to that need.

Even in the home there is much that can be done for boredom. The doctor and nurse will want to review the layout of the sick room, checking whether the patient can see out of the window. They will ensure that, if they can be afforded, there is a television set with remote control, and a radio. Efforts will be made to get the advice of an occupational therapist who is interested in palliative care, or someone talented at advising on creative work such as painting, modelling, writing, and so on. Even a simple roster of visitors helps to bring the world into the patient, but in small doses rather than boluses.

When there is no specific treatment available and the patient is miserable as a result of the increasing weakness and weariness, the doctor and nurse still have something they can offer, something which requires no prescription. They can offer their friendship and their humanity at this, possibly the loneliest time in their patient's life. It might only call for a short phone call to maintain contact or 'dropping in' on the way home at the end of the day.

Special issues in palliative care prescribing

We shall now address some of the therapeutic issues encountered when offering palliative care at home. Though not symptoms they are important and challenging.

Antibiotic use

The mere mention of antibiotics in palliative care produces very polarized views. Some regard their use as medical meddling, officiously striving to keep a person alive, when without the antibiotic the patient would die. They would have a blanket rule—'no antibiotics in palliative care'.

The opposite group would manage every infection as they would at any other time of life. They would identify the offending organism, get sensitivities done, and then treat appropriately even if that meant intravenous administration, regular estimations of plasma levels, hospitalization, and very considerable expense.

There are those who, without thinking what they are saying, speak of pneumonia as 'the old man's friend' as our forefathers used to say. They would probably ask to be placed in the first camp described. Those experienced in modern palliative care would certainly question what sort of friend a patient has in pneumonia!

The fact is that a chest infection, whether or not technically pneumonia, can be very upsetting to the palliative care patient. It produces fever, sweating, dehydration, dry mouth, confusion, and anorexia, to say nothing of the dyspnoea, cough, and offensive sputum which may be difficult to expectorate in their weakened state. To give antibiotics to such a patient can and should be regarded as symptom palliation, not a life-prolonging exercise. The same can be said for infections in the urinary tract.

It would seem to be wise advice:

- to give antibiotics if they can be taken orally and therefore not need hospitalization;
- to check sensitivities if that is feasible;
- never to give antibiotics for a urinary infection in the presence of an indwelling catheter;
- always to explain to relatives (and the patient if able to understand) the rationale behind giving or withholding antibiotics. As we all know most people regard antibiotics as miracle drugs;
- only to give antibiotics if it is thought by doctor and nurse that they will materially contribute to the palliative care/the 'comfort care' of their patient.

Blood transfusion

Iron deficiency anaemia is a feature of almost all life-threatening illness and therefore an obvious feature of the palliative care phase. Its clinical features in no way differ from the condition at other times in life—tiredness, dyspnoea, pallor, drowsiness, confusion, angina, cardiac failure, and palpitations.

In the mind of the layman blood transfusion restores the dying to life. They have seen it for themselves in hospital wards and on television. Some may even have experienced it as patients. Why then is this palliative care patient not being admitted for a blood transfusion when the doctor says his blood is getting weaker?

The following guidelines may help. They apply only to patients receiving palliative care.

- The only symptom which is helped by a transfusion of packed cells (red cell concentrate) is breathlessness. Angina would also improve but few palliative care patients are active enough to be suffering it. It will not improve anything else except perhaps the colour of the patient's cheeks.
- A transfusion should only be given for symptom relief if the haemaglobin (Hb) is lower than 8G.
- Always ask the patient how he/she feels about a repeat transfusion. This is usually very revealing. They often say how much better they felt after the first one several months ago. They looked forward to the same

benefit after the next one but, even though the doctor came and said the post-transfusion blood results were excellent, they did not feel much better. Pressed to say whether they feel it will be worth having another they usually say no, not unless it is certain to make them feel better than they did last time. Time after time patients will agree to a transfusion if it will make either the doctor or the relatives happy!

Both patient and relatives must have all this explained to them. As stated already, they may be puzzled as to why doctors rush to transfuse accident and postoperative patients yet are reluctant to help the palliative care patient. Secretly some wonder if it is because blood is expensive or must be rationed for some reason.

Steroids

Steroids are so valuable in palliative care that one wonders how doctors managed before they were available. Like all useful drugs they have as many adverse effects as they have benefits. Because the patient is in the far-advanced stages of an illness does not absolve the doctor and nurse from weighing in the balance the pros and the cons.

Specific indications

◆ raised intracranial pressure
◆ spinal cord compression
◆ superior vena caval obstruction
◆ extrinsic nerve or nerve root compression

Non-specific indications

◆ anorexia
◆ nausea and vomiting
◆ arthropathies

Drug of choice

Dexamethasone is the drug of choice because the patient has to take fewer tablets than if taking prednisolone or prednisone (dexamethasone 1 milligram equals prednisolone 7 milligrams).

Adverse effects

The principal adverse effects of steroids likely to be encountered in palliative care are as follows.

- Neuropsychiatric: this will usually be mania or hypomania, with euphoria, extreme agitation, flights of fancy, irresponsible and inappropriate behaviour, and sleeplessness. If the dose cannot be reduced the patient must be sedated with chlorpromazine 25–100 milligrams three times a day. Less frequently the drugs will precipitate depression or an agitated anxiety state. Less commonly the patient reports hallucinations and delusions. Hospital admission may be necessary.

- Insomnia: this has been mentioned earlier in this book. It follows on patients taking the drug late in the day. A sedative is rarely needed if the timing of medication is corrected.

- Infection: dormant infection such as tuberculosis can be reactivated and new infections such as candidiasis and pyogenic infections develop yet with little or no fever.

- Voracious appetite: at first exciting to find appetite restored, this soon becomes totally unacceptable and the dose will have to be reduced if possible. Weight increases rapidly even before Cushingoid features show.

- Cushingoid features: this effect is dose and time related. The lower the dose and the shorter the time taking the drug the less the effect and vice versa. It is not totally reversible when the dose is reduced.

- Diabetes mellitus: this occurs in 5–10 per cent of palliative care patients and may present as a subacute diabetic coma easily mistaken for the terminal phase. Dose reduction solves the problem without hypoglycaemics.

- Demineralization: the longer the patient is on steroids the more the osteoporosis will affect the cervical and thoracic spine producing kyphoscoliosis and chronic pain, easily mistaken for the pain of metastases.

- Proximal myopathy: this usually affects the pelvic girdle muscles and less commonly the shoulder and intercostal muscles, the latter leading to difficulties in breathing. Myopathy can be a tragedy for the palliative care patient. His difficulty rising from a chair, getting into a car or bus, even going up and down stairs, is inevitably attributed to the progressive weakness of his underlying illness, rather than the steroids. Unless the drugs are reduced or discontinued the myopathy will not recover.

- Burning perineal pain: this is rare and is said to occur only with the exceedingly high doses of dexamethasone.
- Avascular necrosis of the femoral head is well recognized as a complication but has not been seen by the authors.
- Peptic ulceration: it is doubtful whether steroids alone can produce ulceration. There is, however, no doubt that combining a steroid with an NSAID much increases the risk of ulceration and bleeding. Combining the steroid with an H2 antagonist does not lessen the risk. Combining it with misoprostol or omeprazole does help.

Guidelines for prescribing steroids in palliative care

From the above, certain guidelines can be suggested:

- If possible only prescribe steroids for specific indications
- Prescribe for as short a time as possible keeping the dose as low as possible
- Prescribe with even greater caution if the patient has a history of peptic ulceration, combining the drug with misoprostol or ompeprazole
- Consider the possibility of a dormant infection before prescribing
- Ensure that the dexamethasone is taken early in the day
- Remember to notify any consultants and clinics that steroids have been started.

Fluid replacement

Is there any place for intravenous or subcutaneous infusions when palliative care is being provided at home?

Only a few years ago this question would never have been asked because palliative care was regarded by many as a euphemism for terminal care. Today many patients are very appropriately receiving palliative care at home and are still relatively ambulant, enjoying a social life, and even going on holiday. If they are so 'well' should they not be considered for artificial fluid replacement should the need arise?

We would suggest that intravenous drug infusions should not be set up in a patient's home unless they live far from any hospital. If that is the case there will probably be other factors also suggesting that admission is desirable, even though relatives will have far to travel. It would be unethical to set up an intravenous drip if a professional, whether the nurse or the doctor, could not monitor it as carefully as would happen in a hospital.

Subcutaneous infusion of fluids (hypodermoclysis)

We regard the subcutaneous infusion of fluids such as water or saline as a different matter. The technique is easy and usually without complications. It can be done in the home, does not call for a doctor or nurse to remain in attendance all the time, and can be particularly useful for correcting confusion attributed to dehydration. It can also help relatives who anguish that their loved one is getting insufficient fluids but yet acknowledge that they cannot be taken orally. This is another occasion when it might be helpful to consult a specialist colleague.

Technique

The preferable site is the anterior abdominal wall. An alternative is the anterior axillary fold. It is cleaned in the routine way and a butterfly needle inserted subcutaneously. The infusion set is connected to the needle and the latter kept in place in the usual way with non-allergenic tape. The saline is infused at a rate of 10 drips per minute until 1 litre has been given—the maximum for 24 hours by this route.

If it is thought desirable to aid the local spread of the infused fluid, where the butterfly needle has been inserted one injects hyaluronidase 1500 international units before starting the drip.

Polypharmacy

There is a real danger in palliative care, whether provided in the home or in an in-patient unit, that the patient will become the victim of polypharmacy. He will be put on to a range of medications for his major symptoms, others to deal with their adverse effects, and probably still be on many that he has taken for years.

It has been estimated that the 'average' palliative care patient is on 7.5 different drugs at one time. In a review of 1000 such patients only one was on no medication.

Some questions have to be asked by the prescribing doctor.

1. Which of the drugs the patient has been on for some time need to be continued? It might be possible to discontinue such things as iron preparations, blood pressure lowering agents (advanced disease itself being blood pressure lowering), and 'old timers' such as quinine for night cramps.

2. Can I prescribe for today's problems without having to add in a drug for adverse effects? For example, if a diuretic is required is it possible

to use potassium sparing one? Is there an analgesic that will not need an adjuvant laxative?

3. Can the regimen be simplified? Can this cough be relieved without more oral medication? Rather than 4 hourly medication can I now make it 12 or 24 hourly? Does the patient need both an antidepressant and a sedative or could one drug deal with both? Why does the patient need enemata as well as oral laxatives?

As at all times in palliative care these discussions should be between doctor and nurse, their decisions be recorded in the notes, and everything explained not only to the patient but to the relatives.

The logic of them will, at first, be obvious to the relatives. It is, after all, they who probably have to count out the pills and tablets, persuade the frail patient to take them, and who may sometimes themselves be confused by them all. What they will not find so easy to accept is that some of the long-standing prescriptions are to be discontinued. 'The specialist said he would have to take them all his life and here are you stopping them' or 'Whenever he forgot to take that one he got angina so why are you stopping it?' This topic is discussed in Chapter 13 on 'the final days'.

Finally, it cannot be overstated that a simple drug/medication chart is indispensable. It helps the doctor and nurse when they visit the patient. It helps colleagues who are standing in for the regular doctor and nurse. It explains to relatives what to give and why. It can be taken to hospital clinics and should always be taken to the hospice or specialist palliative care unit when the patient is admitted. Until such time as we all use Patient Held Records, the palliative care medication charts will be the next best thing.

3

Pain palliation

Many patients with cancer believe pain to be an inevitable consequence of their diagnosis. Although pain is one of the most common symptoms, occurring in about 80 per cent of patients with advanced cancer, the majority of pains can be controlled by implementing simple guidelines. However, patients often remember examples of terrible suffering in a family member or a close friend. Why is it that doctors fail to control pain when effective analgesics exist? The possible reasons for failure to relieve pain include:

- failure to assess and establish a cause for the pain
- failure to take into account social, psychological, and spiritual components of the pain
- waiting for the patient to complain of pain and thus failing ever to catch up with the pain
- inadequate doses for breakthrough pain
- lack of use of co-analgesics
- lack of experience in titrating drugs to match the level of pain
- withholding strong opioids because of misplaced fears of addiction, respiratory depression, and tolerance, or of shortening the patient's life
- failure to think of disease-modifying therapies such as radiotherapy, chemotherapy, surgery, or hormone therapy
- lack of use of nerve blocks and spinal analgesia
- failure to review regularly the symptom control
- failure to seek specialist advice when simple measures fail
- failure to provide clear instructions for drug regimens
- failure to set realistic goals in partnership with patients and their families.

The principles of pain control

- Assess the cause of each pain. Remember that most patients will have several different pains. These may be due to the cancer and its metastases, or treatment related, for example postoperative adhesions or associated conditions such as constipation or pressure sores. Pre-existing conditions such as osteoarthritis can account for up to 25 per cent of pains.

- Address total pain. Pain has social, psychological, spiritual, and psychological elements in addition to the physical causes.

- Set realistic goals—involve the patient and relatives in decision making.

- Use the analgesic ladder and co-analgesics.

- Give regular analgesia titrated to relieve pain.

- Have confidence in the oral route.

- Explain as much as they want to know to the patient and family.

- Review frequently.

- Empathy, understanding, and relief of fear are essential. An interested doctor or nurse is a powerful analgesic.

Types of pain

Cancer pains may be broadly divided into two types: nociceptive, resulting from tissue injury; and neuropathic, due to nerve injury.

Nociceptive pain

Nociceptive pains include the following important groups:

1. *Visceral pain* may be produced by tumour in the liver, spleen, or kidney causing capsular stretching. It is described as a sickening, dull, deep-seated ache over the affected organ, made worse on palpation. Pain may also result from tumour involvement of the parietal peritoneum or from perforation of a hollow viscus. Partial or complete obstruction of bowel, ureter, or bladder may cause distension and muscle spasm. Colic is described as intermittent, short-lived recurrent pain, which builds up to a crescendo.

2. *Bone pain* may be due to metastases, osteoporosis, vertebral collapse or fractures. A fracture or collapse should be suspected when severe pain develops acutely in an area clearly localized by the patient. Metastatic bone pain may be described as a dull, aching pain and may

be accompanied by localized bony tenderness. Incident pain is precipitated by weight bearing or movement in patients with bone metastases. It may occur when pain at rest is well controlled and can present a difficult management challenge.

3. *Muscular pains* may be accompanied by tender trigger points which may be palpated and localized to a fingertip.

4. *Headache* may be due to cerebral oedema, a primary or secondary brain tumour, or skull bone metastases. Cancer patients may also suffer headaches from any of the various non-malignant causes of headache.

Neuropathic pain

Neuropathic pain results from damage to nerve tissue either by tumour infiltration or by tumour compression. It may also be a consequence of treatment, for example radiotherapy, chemotherapy, or surgery, or arise from a coexisting condition such as a viral infection.

Neuropathic pain is pain or aching felt in an area of altered sensation. Aching may be severe. The pain may be described as shooting or burning, with a background severe ache or terrible discomfort. The patient may also describe areas of numbness which are tender to touch, pins and needles or pain caused by non-painful stimuli such as light touch or cold (allodynia).

Classically the patient is uncomfortable at rest, clutching or rubbing the affected limb in an attempt to relieve the excruciating aching pain.

Cancer pain management: general principles

The analgesic ladder

The World Health Organization's three-step analgesic ladder (Fig. 3.1) remains the gold standard of the use of analgesic drugs in cancer pain. If it is used correctly it is effective. Have no fear of tolerance, addiction, or respiratory depression but become confident in using this simple guide to effective pain relief.

Co-analgesics (or adjuvants) are drugs which are not analgesics in themselves but work with analgesics to contribute to effective analgesia.

Using the ladder

Step 1—non-opioids (e.g. paracetamol): the patient is prescribed paracetamol 1 gram four times a day regularly by mouth. When pain persists or increases the doctor moves to *Step 2*.

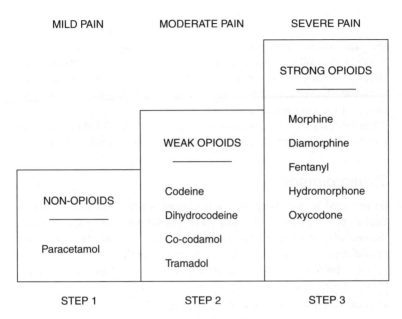

Fig. 3.1 WHO analgesic ladder.

Step 2—weak opioids (e.g. compound drugs containing codeine): there is little to choose between these *Step 2* analgesics. The patient is prescribed one regularly orally so long as pain is controlled. When pain control is lost, there is nothing to be gained by changing to another *Step 2* analgesic and the doctor must move to *Step 3*. A common reason for inadequate pain relief is a doctor's reluctance to move to *Step 3*. The decision to move to a strong opioid depends on the severity of pain not on the length of prognosis.

Step 3—strong opioids (e.g. morphine): starting with rapid-release oral morphine 5–10 milligrams every 4 hours. This acts within 20 minutes and provides analgesia for 4 hours. The dose is titrated up until pain is controlled. Extra doses of the same amount are prescribed for break-through pain as often as necessary. If breakthrough doses have been required then the regular 4 hourly dose is increased to account for this the following day.

When the pain is well controlled, the rapid-release 4-hourly morphine may be converted to a twice-daily sustained-release tablet. Rapid-release morphine must still be available for breakthrough pain. There is no maximum dose for morphine so long as the drug is having an effect on the pain. Whereas most patients will be satisfactorily pain controlled on less than 200 milligrams of oral morphine a day, a few (particularly young adults) will need very much larger doses. If the dose needs to be increased to high levels over a few days, it may be helpful to discuss the pain management with a specialist colleague.

Lower doses may be adequate in patients with renal failure, as active metabolites of morphine may accumulate if renal function is poor.

Strong opioids

Be prepared to use morphine early if pain is not controlled at *Step 2*. Explain to the patient and family about regular 4-hourly administration, the necessity of recording breakthrough medication, that there is no risk of addiction, and that morphine does not hasten death.

Warn about important persisting side-effects and some which may be transient. Common side-effects of morphine are:

* constipation—always prescribe a laxative;
* nausea—consider haloperidol 1.5 milligrams at night for 5 nights;
* drowsiness—may be a sign of overdosage;
* dry mouth—mouth care.

Less common side-effects of morphine are:

* itching, sweats, and confusion.

Titration

Use an oral rapid-acting morphine preparation which commences action in 20 minutes and lasts 4 hours, increasing the dose by 30–50 per cent if pain occurs.

Once stable pain control has been achieved then convert the 4-hourly dose to twice daily sustained-release morphine. For example: 20 milligrams rapid-release morphine 4 hourly = 120 milligrams morphine daily = 60 milligrams sustained-release twice daily.

Breakthrough pain

Use rapid-acting oral morphine prescribing one-sixth of the total daily dose as often as required to relieve breakthrough pain.

Alternative routes of administration

Although morphine is available in suppository form, most patients find a syringe driver more convenient to use if the oral route is not feasible for reasons such as vomiting, dysphagia, confusion, or coma.

Diamorphine is the preferred opioid for injections and for the syringe driver because of its excellent solubility. Oral diamorphine should not be used. Table 3.1 gives the guidelines for drug compatibility with diamorphine in syringe drivers.

Converting oral morphine to subcutaneous diamorphine

The total daily dose of oral morphine should be divided by 3 to give the 24-hour total dose of diamorphine in the syringe driver.

For example: 90 milligrams sustained-release morphine twice daily = 180 milligrams daily oral morphine = 60 milligrams subcutaneous diamorphine over 24 hours in the syringe driver.

If injections of diamorphine are required for breakthrough pain then one-sixth of the total daily dose in the syringe driver may be given.

For example: the patient receiving 60 milligrams diamorphine subcutaneously over 24 hours via syringe driver would need 10 milligrams diamorphine for breakthrough pain, given as often as needed, even hourly, until the pain is brought under control.

Alternative opioids

Morphine and diamorphine are the first-line strong opioids for cancer pain. However, uncommonly, the side-effects can be so troublesome that there is a need to change to an alternative opioid which may also have side-effects but be better tolerated by the patient. It is important to be sure that you are dealing with a pain which is responsive to opioids and that an adjuvant analgesic is not indicated. This is often a complex situation where discussion with specialist colleagues is indicated.

Fentanyl

A strong opioid administered by a transdermal patch which lasts 3 days. Fentanyl patches are long-acting preparations and are thus not suitable for titration in a situation where pain control is not stable and the opioid requirement has not been determined.

Table 3.1 Guidelines for drug compatibility with diamorphine in syringe drivers

Drug	BNF Ref.	Presentation	Usual daily dose	Indication	Compatibility with diamorphine	Comments
Cyclizine	4.6	50 mg/ml	150 mg	Antiemetic in intestinal obstruction Raised I.C.P.	Above 10 mg/ml cyclizine may precipitate	Do not dilute with sodium chloride 0.9% May precipitate with dexamethasone
Haloperidol	4.2.1	5 mg/ml	2.5–5 mg for nausea 5–20 mg for sedation	First-line antiemetic for drug-induced and metabolic nausea	Haloperidol 4 mg/ml compatible with diamorphine up 50 mg/ml Haloperidol 3 mg/ml compatible with diamorphine up to 100 mg/ml	Do not use oily depot injection Consider single daily injection
Hyoscine butylbromide (Buscopan)	1.2	20 mg/ml	Colic 60–120 mg Bronchial hypersecretion 20 mg stat, then 20 mg/24 h	Colic Bronchial hypersecretion	Hyoscine butylbromide 20 mg/ml compatible with diamorphine up to 150 mg/ml	Butylbromide less sedative than hydrobromide May precipitate with cyclizine
Methotrimeprazine (Nozinan)	4.2.1	25 mg/ml	25–200 mg 12.5–25 mg (if sedation not required)	Antiemetic if agitation also present Low-dose antiemetic without sedation	Compatible at usual doses Reconstitute diamorphine + further dilute, with sodium chloride 0.9%	May cause lumps at infusion site. If so, dilute further Consider use of single injection 12.5 mg subcutaneously at night for nausea
Metocloramide	4.6	10 mg/2 ml	30–60 mg Higher doses may be used, seek specialist advice	Non-sedating antiemetic	Metoclopramide 5 mg/ml compatible with diamorphine up to 150 mg/ml	May cause extra-pyramidal side-effects in young patients Avoid in GI obstruction with colic

Drug	BNF ref	Concentration	Starting dose	Indication	Syringe driver compatibility	Notes
Midazolam	15.1.4	10 mg/2 ml	10–120 mg starting dose from 10 mg	Control of terminal restlessness Convulsions	Midazolam 5 mg/ml compatible with diamorphine up to 33 mg/ml	Useful if patient 'jerky', has Parkinson's, or is prone to seizures

Specialist use only

Drug	BNF ref	Concentration	Starting dose	Indication	Syringe driver compatibility	Notes
Octreotide	8.3.4.3	50 µg/ml 100 µg/ml 500 µg/ml 1 mg/5 ml	300–600 µg	Antiemetic in intestinal obstruction Diarrhoea In fistulae	Contact Drug Information	Incompatible with cyclizine
Ondansetron	4.6	4 mg/2 ml 8 mg/4 ml	16 mg	Antiemetic acting on 5HT3 receptor	Contact Drug Information	Use if other antiemetics have failed
Ketamine	15.1.1	100 mg/ml	100–300 mg/24 h	Neuropathic pain	Separate syringe driver	
Ketorolac	15.1.4.2	10 mg/ml 30 mg/ml	60–90 mg	Strong NSAID	Contact Drug Information	Dilute in sodium chloride 0.9% Precipitates with cyclizine Separate syringe driver May cause GI bleeding
Phenobarbitone	4.8.1		200–800 mg	Convulsions and severe terminal agitation	Not compatible Must have separate syringe driver	

Note: dexamethasone injection 4 mg/ml usual daily dose 4–16 mg may be given as a single injection rather than in a syringe driver (BNF Ref. 6.3.2).

The following drugs should NEVER be used in the syringe driver: diazepam; prochlorperazine; chlorpromazine.

Stability of drug mixtures for subcutaneous infusion

The drugs have been documented as being physically and chemically stable with diamorphine. For advice on mixing more than two drugs seek specialist advice.

Reconstitute diamorphine and further dilute with water except when to be mixed with ketorolac or methotrimeprazine (Nozinan) when sodium chloride 0.9% should be used.

Use combinations within 24 hours of mixing.

Visually inspect the mixture for signs of precipitation at regular intervals, particularly at high doses.

Indications for a fentanyl patch

Fentanyl is an alternative for patients whose pain is under control and for whom the opioid responsiveness has been determined by titration. If pain levels are stable fentanyl offers an alternative to morphine:

◆ when the oral route is no longer feasible;

◆ if constipation with morphine has been difficult to control despite appropriate laxative use;

◆ in patients who cannot comply with twice daily sustained-release morphine.

It should not be used in opioid naïve patients or in cases of acute pain.

Although constipation is less of a problem than with morphine, laxatives are often needed. Some patients may experience morphine withdrawal symptoms when changed from oral morphine to fentanyl patches. These symptoms are transient and are treated by giving an appropriate breakthrough dose of oral morphine.

Morphine or diamorphine should be prescribed for breakthrough pain in addition to the fentanyl patch. In a terminally ill patient fentanyl patches should be continued and additional diamorphine titrated by injection and then added to a syringe driver.

To calculate a breakthrough dose of subcutaneous diamorphine, divide the patch strength by 5 and give this dose in milligrams of diamorphine subcutaneous.stat.

For example: 50 micrograms an hour fentanyl patch = 10 milligrams breakthrough dose of diamorphine.

Hydromorphone

Hydromorphone is about seven times as potent as morphine. Rapid-acting tablets which last 4 hours and a 12-hourly slow-release capsule are available. For example: 1.3 milligrams rapid-acting hydromorphone = 10 milligrams rapid-acting oral morphine solution. Side-effects are similar to morphine but it may be more useful in patients with renal failure.

Methadone

Methadone is available in tablet and injection form. It has an unpredictable half-life which may lead to accumulation of the drug. It should be reserved for specialist use only.

Opioid toxicity

The ability of patients to tolerate opioids depends upon many factors: renal function, speed of dose escalation, opioid sensitivity of pain, age, and other medication. Hepatic dysfunction is not important, and jaundiced patients may be given opioids. Opioid toxicity may present as:

- agitation
- confusion with hallucinations
- myoclonic jerks
- slowed respiration
- pinpoint pupils
- coma.

If the agitated confusion is mistaken as a symptom of pain, further opioids may be given with a worsening of the situation.

Treatment involves reducing the opioids, using adjuvant analgesics, and then possibly retitrating with an alternative opioid. Haloperidol may be useful to control agitation. If alternative opioids are considered, this is a time to seek specialist advice.

In severe cases of opioid toxicity naloxone may have to be administered intravenously to reverse life-threatening toxicity, making this a real ethical dilemma.

Opioid responsiveness

Not all pains respond to opioids. It is probably better to think in terms of a spectrum of responsiveness. At one end would be the highly responsive visceral pains and, at the other, the much less responsive neuropathic pains. In the middle lie bone pains. It is always worth a trial of a titration with morphine before making any assumptions about degree of responsiveness.

Adjuvant analgesics, radiotherapy, nerve blocks, and spinal anaesthetics may need to be considered if pains are not relieved by opioids.

Challenging pains

The general principles of pain management and the use of opioids have been described. They apply whatever the cause and site of pain. However, certain specific pains require specific treatments in addition.

Bone pain

Remember that bone pain is only partially opioid sensitive. Incident (movement-related) pain may be a problem. Paracetamol 1G four times a day may be more effective than increasing the morphine if the latter is having no beneficial effect. Incident pain may be helped by giving rapid-release morphine 20 minutes before movements which precipitate pain rather than increasing the slow-acting 12-hourly morphine with resultant oversedation at rest. In managing bone pain co-analgesics such as non-steroidal anti-inflammatory drugs (NSAIDs) may be beneficial and palliative radiotherapy may bring dramatic relief. It is sometimes helpful to consider specialist advice regarding spinal routes of administration of analgesics in this situation.

Non-steroidal anti-inflammatory drugs (NSAIDs)

These work as inhibitors of cyclo-oxygenase enzymes (COX inhibitors). COX1 causes the gastric and renal side-effects while COX2 is responsible for the anti-inflammatory actions. Most widely used NSAIDS have both COX1 and 2 effects, although newer drugs such as meloxicam and rofe-coxib are claimed to be more COX2 selective. There is insufficient evidence at present, in patients with advanced cancer and bone metastases, to substantiate anecdotal case reports.

It is probably best to familiarize yourself with a few NSAIDs, for example:

- ibuprofen 400–600 milligrams three times a day (maximum 2.4 grams daily), low risk of gastrointestinal (GI) bleeding;
- diclofenac 75 milligrams twice a day (maximum licensed in BNF 150 milligrams a day but sometimes 100 milligrams twice a day needed for bone pain), intermediate risk of GI bleed;
- piroxicam 20 milligrams daily: the melt formulation may be helpful if swallowing is difficult, higher risk of GI bleed, use with caution in the elderly;
- lansoprazole 30 milligrams daily: gastric protection is indicated in the following situations:
  - history of peptic ulcer
  - over 70 years old
  - concomitant steroid therapy.

Palliative radiotherapy

Patients suspected of bone metastases need early referral to a clinical oncologist. Bone pain is the commonest indication for radiotherapy.

Radiotherapy is highly effective in palliating bone pain. The dose is often only a single fraction. Side-effects are generally nausea and tiredness, and pain may initially be exacerbated. Pain relief is variable in onset; some patients seem to feel a benefit within days while others may need to wait 4–6 weeks before feeling the full benefit. When this relief is obtained, the dose of opioid may often be reduced. This is a reminder that pain is a physiological antagonist to opioids. As pain is reduced by another modality (radiotherapy), there is relatively an excess of opioid and the patient feels drowsy and gets pin-point pupils—signs of toxicity which call for dose reduction.

Oncologists will be involved in decisions about palliative radiotherapy. The general practitioner is well placed to be involved in discussions on further disease-modifying chemotherapy or hormone therapy, often being better placed to discuss issues of quality of life with the patient.

Other measures to discuss with the specialist team when managing difficult bone pain are:

♦ *Bisphosphonates*: in addition to their role in the management of hypercalcaemia and myeloma, bisphosphonates may also be effective in relieving bone pain, particularly in patients with widespread bone metastases who are unable to receive further radiotherapy yet are normocalcaemic. Patients with bone metastases from breast cancer, prostatic cancer, and myeloma are the commonest groups to benefit. The treatment is best given as an intravenous infusion of sodium pamidronate on an in-patient or day-case basis.

♦ *Steroids*: dexamethasone 2–12 milligrams a day may help to give temporary relief from pain.

♦ *Spinal analgesia and nerve blocks*: particularly in patients with difficult incident pain, these techniques should be discussed with an anaesthetist.

♦ *Orthopaedic interventions*: stabilization of fractures, long bones, spine and joint replacements are palliative interventions which may have to be considered even when disease is advanced.

♦ *Physiotherapy and occupational therapy*: as in all palliative care, a multidisciplinary team approach is essential. Nowhere is this better demonstrated than in the rehabilitation of patients with advanced cancer with limited mobility and pain due to bone metastases. Physiotherapists and occupational therapists work with the patient and family to maximize functional ability and to provide advice on how to cope best with the everyday activities of living at home.

Visceral pain

Visceral pain responds well to use of the analgesic ladder. Co-analgesics have a place in specific situations. In liver capsule pain dexamethasone 4–12 milligrams a day acts as a co-analgesic. The dose may be reduced once the pain has settled. Some difficult cases may benefit from a coeliac plexus block. Pain due to pancreatic or gastric cancer may respond well to a coeliac axis block if conventional use of the analgesic ladder fails to relieve pain. It is helpful to discuss these management problems with a specialist at an early stage when difficulties in pain control are first encountered.

Colic due to subacute intestinal obstruction responds well to hyoscine butylbromide, which is most effective given by the subcutaneous route either 20 milligrams three times a day or 60–120 milligrams over 24 hours via a syringe driver. Hyoscine butylbromide may also help to relieve the pains of bladder spasms and ureteric pain.

Neuropathic pain

Neuropathic pain is usually only partially responsive to opioids. Indeed, it is often the poor response to opioids which alerts the doctor to the presence of neuropathic pain. However, it is worthwhile titrating with a strong opioid in the usual manner described above, to determine whether it confers any benefit. Control of the pain will usually depend on the use of co-analgesics.

Co-analgesics in neuropathic pain

Tricyclic antidepressants

Amitriptyline is the tricyclic antidepressant of choice in the treatment of neuropathic pain. The starting dose is 25 milligrams (10 milligrams in the elderly). The dose may be increased every 5 days, a response usually being achieved in the dose range 25–75 milligrams. Side-effects include a dry mouth, blurred vision, constipation, and sedation. Although the newer selective serotonin uptake inhibitors have fewer side-effects, they do not relieve neuropathic pain. If there is an inadequate response or if side-effects limit dose titration or if there is a lancinating component to the pain then add an anticonvulsant.

Anticonvulsants

Start with a low dose and titrate upwards. There are several anticonvulsants which act as co-analgesics.

- Sodium valproate 200 milligrams twice a day up to 1600 milligrams a day maximum.
- Carbamazepine 200 milligrams a day up to 400 milligrams twice a day maximum. Hypotension and dizziness may limit its use.
- Clonazepam 0.5 milligrams nocte up to 2 milligrams a day maximum. Sedation may be a problem.
- Gabapentin is a more recent drug used for neuropathic pain. Its use should be discussed with a specialist.

Corticosteroids in neuropathic pain

Dexamethasone 8 milligrams a day taken before midday may reduce perineural oedema and nerve compression. If there is no improvement within 2 or 3 days the drug may be stopped. If there is an improvement then the dose should be reduced by 2 milligrams a week to the lowest dose which helps to relieve pain.

Measures requiring specialist advice in neuropathic pain

Anti-arrhythmic drugs

- Mexiletine 50–100 milligrams three times a day may be used if tricyclics and anticonvulsants have failed to relieve pain. Higher doses may be needed with specialist advice.
- Flecainide is an alternative.

Ketamine

Ketamine may be given by subcutaneous infusion via a syringe driver. It acts as an N-Methyl D-Aspartate (NMDA) receptor antagonist. Ketamine should not be used if there is a history of raised intracranial pressure or fits. It can cause hallucinations and confusion.

Non-drug methods of analgesia

Transcutaneous electrical nerve stimulation

This acts on the large A fibres and controls pain by 'closing the gate'. Advice can be obtained from physiotherapists, specialist palliative care nurses, or from the pain clinic on the positioning of the electrodes.

Acupuncture

Some patients are keen to pursue this form of complementary therapy. It is best provided by a skilled therapist working in conjunction with the pain team.

Radiotherapy

Palliative radiotherapy, in addition to its key role in relieving the pain of bone metastases, may help to induce tumour shrinkage and relieve nerve compression.

The pain team

Nowhere is a close liaison between the general practitioner, palliative care specialist, and anaesthetist more important than in the management of neuropathic pain. If conservative methods outlined above fail to control pain or if side-effects become too troublesome then we need to consider either a spinal route of drug administration, a nerve block, or nerve destruction.

Neuropathic pain is often difficult to control since it takes time for the various co-analgesics to take effect. Time needs to be spent with the patient and relatives at the outset in acknowledging these difficulties and in setting realistic goals. Pain relief results from a multidisciplinary approach including nurses, doctors, physiotherapists, occupational therapists, and often the wider pain team.

If pain is not responding satisfactorily what does the GP do next?

When the patient continues to complain of pain the doctor and nurse need to ask the following questions:

♦ Has the pain, or pains, been correctly diagnosed?
♦ Are the correct drugs being taken at the correct dose at the right intervals?

- Is the pain responsive to opioids?
- Is the pain responding to the drugs prescribed?
- Is there a new pain and if so what is causing it?
- Have we addressed emotional, spiritual, and social factors?
- Have we carefully reviewed the patient?
- Have we discussed the management with the rest of the team?
- Should we discuss this case with a specialist colleague?

4
___

Psychosocial issues

In this chapter we shall look at the apprehensions, anxieties, and emotional upheavals experienced by the patient, the kaleidoscope of emotions felt by the relatives and friends and, finally, how they affect each other. We recognize how artificial it is to separate the problems of the patient from those of the relatives but will do so here merely to make presentation easier.

Uncertainties for patients

Experience shows that most people coming to the end of life have many uncertainties and fears even when they claim to be ready 'to go', have a strong faith, and a caring family. For the doctor and nurse the important thing to remember is that patients may not express these uncertainties unless given the opportunity and even some encouragement to do so. We have come to appreciate that just because someone does not mention they have pain does not mean they have no pain! It only means they did not speak about it. The same applies to many of the fears and apprehensions these patients have. They may be deeply upset or frightened about their illness or its treatment but not mention that to either the doctor or the nurse. Once again it is worth emphasizing that terminally ill people choose who they will say things to. They may speak of breathlessness to the doctor and never mention any other anxieties, but tell the nurse all about their fears of choking to death. Only when the doctor and the other members of the primary care team share their knowledge, does the whole picture emerge.

Patients may be apprehensive of:

1. Pain and other symptoms either not being recognized and taken seriously by the doctor or being inadequately treated. It is a truism that palliative care patients stop reporting symptoms when no one seems to recognize how much they are suffering or their medication is not

changed to bring the problems under better control. It must also be remembered that these patients do not expect medication for each symptom but they do want it to be known that they have the problem which may call for treatment later.

2. The things all human beings fear, namely death from haemorrhage, choking, or asphyxia. No matter how unlikely any of these are, the patient needs to be reassured. When the doctor or nurse says nothing, it only adds to the patient's anxieties because they assume their fears are well founded. For example, they are not helped when a doctor looks at the fleck of blood in a sputum cup and fails to say that that is a common thing which does not herald a big, possibly catastrophic bleed. The motor neurone disease patient understandably expects to die 'fighting for breath' but can be truthfully reassured that that does not happen because before then he gets sleepier and unaware of what is happening.

3. Increasing dependency, necessitating help with toileting, bathing, even feeding and moving around in bed. When people learn they have a fatal illness, particularly cancer, they expect loss of weight and are certain they will have pain but few seem to realize they will become so dependent. It can be very distressing for them. It is made worse by the feeling that not only are they dependent and 'a burden' but that they are not needed by anyone, that they are now useless. There is no prescription for this, only the genuine understanding and respect of the doctor and nurse.

4. The frailer they get the more they sense the tiredness and grief of the family, the tensions and the occasional tears. Given the chance, they speak to the doctor and nurse about their fears for the family's future, the income, the rent or the mortgage, the house, the schooling for the grandchildren, and so forth. There is no doubt, as we have said elsewhere in this book, that an important and common reason for someone agreeing to be admitted to a hospital or hospice is because of the burden they feel they are on the family members. They need to be most strongly reassured, in a way that the family doctor can in his or her unique role, that the family left behind will still be cherished and cared for.

5. Particularly when the patient is in hospital or likely to be readmitted there, they fear further investigations which they sense may not make any difference to their care or their prognosis. They have seen it happen in the past that they know how often doctors request X-rays and blood

tests rather than sitting down to explain things to them, and then fail to tell the patient the results of the tests. This anxiety must be addressed and also reported to hospital colleagues.

6. Obvious as it may sound, our patients fear the unknown. Whatever experiences they have had in life, whatever coping skills they have developed, dying is something they have never done before. Understandably, they wonder what has been kept back from them, what new pains they might experience, how much they may have to suffer, who will be with them, and so forth. The only way to help them is to reassure that they will never be left alone, that everyone is being totally honest with them, and that everything that can be done will be done to help them.

7. Abandonment. Patients worry in case their doctors and nurses will no longer be interested in them as their condition deteriorates, will not visit them so frequently, or will have them admitted because they need so much time and attention. Paradoxically, some patients wonder if this is why admission to a hospice or specialist palliative care unit is being suggested for them.

Uncertainties for relatives

Again, something which seems so obvious: the uncertainties, fears, and apprehensions of the relatives are not the same as the patient's. It is quite possible to give good care to the patient and overlook the needs of the relatives and other carers. A widow, reflecting on her husband's care, told one of the authors how wonderfully he had cared for her late husband. Before he could say a word she told him that at times she felt she hated him, their doctor of several years: 'You used to come in, sit and talk with him, make him laugh like old times then run downstairs where all you did was put an arm round my shoulder and tell me I was doing a wonderful job. When did you ever ask if I was sleeping well, how I was feeling, if I was terrified about the future? Not once! I needed someone to be interested in me as well as in my husband.'

Their anxieties can be divided into those relating to the patient (which they are happy to talk about) and those more related to their own needs (which they may never speak of unless encouraged to do so). Obviously they are closely, inextricably related.

Related to the patient

♦ Almost all 'lay' carers feel inadequate for the task of caring at home. As they often point out they have not done it before and have had no training. This sense of inadequacy is something the professionals should bear in mind. Most people reach their middle years before having a death in the family, attending a funeral, or seeing a mortally ill person. Many can go through their whole life without seeing a dead body. The only deaths they have witnessed are those on film or television. Is it any wonder they are apprehensive. To add to this anxiety they suspect that it takes great skills and experience to be able to care properly if doctors have to become specialists in palliative medicine, nurses have to take additional diplomas, and special units have to be built, all to look after the terminally ill.

They are anxious about oral hygiene, moving the patient in bed, helping him to the toilet, helping with feeding, bathing, dressing, and even walking. All these skills can be taught by the nurse as part of her contribution to palliative care in the home.

♦ Particularly if they have tried to shield the patient from the truth (usually unsuccessfully) they dread having to answer difficult questions or having to cope with tears, anger, guilt, or any of the myriad emotions experienced by the patient and family at this time. The doctor will, of course, explain that honesty is the only course of action and will be demonstrating that in his dealings with the patient, but that may not help the wife or husband who has so vehemently denied to the patient (and even themselves) that death was inevitable.

It is important for the doctor and nurse to demonstrate the skill of finding out exactly what the patient and nearest relative knows and, usually a different thing, how each wants to deal with that information. We must recognize two different scenarios here.

Both husband and wife (for example) may know the diagnosis and prognosis, and also know that the other knows everything. However, each elects to speak and behave as though neither of them knows anything. Provided this does not prevent them speaking about it if one has to, or in other ways acknowledging it, this does not matter. The doctor and nurse can feel safe joining in this loving conspiracy.

The more dangerous scenario is when one or other, or both, know everything there is to be known about the tragic situation but continue to speak and act as though nothing was wrong. They go to elaborate lengths to deny the reality of what is happening, telling complicated lies, planning holidays, ordering clothes, forbidding anyone (including doctors, nurses, clergy, and friends) from speaking about the illness. This is dangerous and counter-productive because both patient and relative are prevented from verbalizing concerns, asking questions, putting their affairs in order, repairing relationships, and getting closer to each other and those they love. Here the doctor and nurse must make it clear that although they understand why they are behaving in this way, they will not be party to it because it is not in the best interest of either the patient or the relatives.

Equally important is that the patient is constantly reassured that there is no talking behind his back or on the doorstep, no conspiracy between the relatives and professionals. Contentment needs honesty and cannot coexist with secrecy.

- Research has shown that relatives often perceive the patient as suffering more pain and anxiety than is actually the case. No matter how much the patient protests she slept well, has no pain, and feels very comfortable, the relatives will urge the doctor not to listen to her. She is, they say, suffering terribly and too brave to admit it. This must be seen as them protecting the loved one, acting as advocate between the patient and the sceptics. They must be encouraged to discuss everything with the patient, be taught things they can do to help, and to keep a written record of their concerns which can then be raised later with the health professional.

- People fear that they will not know when the patient is dying or be able to recognize when death has occurred. Experience shows that time spend describing everything is never wasted—colour changes, Cheyne–Stokes respiration, the 'death rattle', changes in temperature of the limbs, etc. It is also useful to explain that even the unconscious person is probably able to hear things said at the bedside. Relatives will want to know what to do at the time of death, whether to move the patient, when to phone the doctor, and where.

- Finally, in relation to the patient, relatives have to live day in, day out, with the advice gratuitously offered by all and sundry. Friends and neighbours suggest or comment on where the patient should be cared for, who the best doctor is, what new treatment they have heard is available in the United States, and so forth. They never seem to go anywhere without a neighbour, a friend from church, or a fellow-shopper in the supermarket offering them unsolicited advice or criticism. The only answer is the sense of safety and reassurance they get from the professional confidence and team-working of the doctor and nurse. Consistency of advice is critically important at this time. Even a hint of disagreement between the professional carers can be most damaging.

Related to themselves

In a nutshell, the immediate family and friends are trying to cope with the practicalities of caring whilst, at the same time, grieving and looking forward to a very different future. They can speak of today's caring but it feels indecent to talk of their grief and tomorrow's problems when their loved one is still alive in the next room.

+ They are usually concerned about their own health, and often with good reason. They may be elderly themselves and not enjoying good health. They have usually programmed themselves to care for a limited time and are anxious and embarrassed when the patient lives on beyond what they were led to expect. This is particularly a problem when good palliative care is provided. Without pain and with so much effort and attention being put into raising the quality of life, palliative care patients seem to live much longer than anyone expected. It cannot be urged strongly enough that both the doctor and nurse set aside a few minutes at each visit to ask about the carers and ensure than everything is being done to keep them well. This is where a Palliative Care Day Unit is a godsend—it gives them a break for a few hours and they can be confident that the patient is being well cared for and enjoying themselves.

+ They may dread the future for a variety of reasons—loneliness, reduced income, different way of life without a partner, having to do 'the business of the house' which the spouse had always done, meeting people in the street, and so forth. The list is endless. Simply acknowledging these fears and offering to help, or get in someone who can help, is usually sufficient. Most people cope better than they ever thought possible.

+ More delicate and difficult is the not-uncommon situation when the surviving spouse is not grieving for one reason or another. The illness may have been so protracted that the grieving was done long ago. The patient may have had a personality change so that the spouse feels he/she is not the person they married and loved. The patient may have been unconscious for some time during which the spouse or partner came to terms with their loss and new situation. Much more common is the couple who would have divorced long ago had it not been for the mortal illness. The healthy one remained to care for the spouse whom they had long stopped loving. To cry and behave like a grieving partner would be impossible, especially when (as they may whisper to the doctor or nurse) they look forward to the death as a release and as a chance to start a new life. All of these scenarios call for a good listening ear and empathetic nod of agreement. Nothing more.

◆ Many are apprehensive about making funeral arrangements and how to meet the expenses. They assume that it is a complicated business and are reassured when the doctor in less than five minutes explains the routine, what things they need to discuss and decide in advance, and what certificates will be asked for. The doctor need never be apprehensive about talking about death and what to do. Experience has shown that relatives find it reassuring.

◆ Reference has already been made in this book to the uncomfortable, distressing emotions experienced when a loved ones is dying; emotions such as anger against the medical profession, against society, or even against God; guilt about past events or relationships; bitterness, resentments, hopelessness, regrets. It can be a veritable kaleidoscope, outside anyone's control, serving no purpose, exhausting, and often frightening. It is useful when a doctor feels there is more going on in the mind and heart of the closest relative or friend than he can fathom, to invite them to unburden themselves. 'This is a time when you feel overwhelmed with so many different feelings, don't you? You cannot make sense of things. Would it help if you poured them out on me? I've time to listen if you think it might help.' It does help and usually does not take as much time as you expected!

Family differences

The cynic has remarked that 'where there is a Will there is a fray'. Problems usually arise long before the reading of the Will, however. They are often the most testing feature of palliative care, whether in the home or in a hospice or palliative care unit.

What usually happens is that distant relatives arrive on the scene. Little may have been heard of them or from them for years. Now they 'take over', demanding to see the doctors, questioning if the best treatment has been given, and asking why other specialists have not been called in. The immediate relatives who have had all the anxieties and done all the caring in recent months or years are ignored as if they do not exist. Soon tensions

lead to open disagreements and disputes. In no time it looks like a dysfunctional family, all with separate opinions, all criticizing each other, the
patient often spoken about but almost ignored, the grieving spouse left
to feel more helpless and bereft than ever. To be fair it also has to be
admitted that most people do not find it easy to understand explanations
given by doctors, and therefore relatives may have found it difficult keeping
distant family members accurately informed.

It is tempting for the doctor to drop any hopes of caring for the person
at home and to arrange hospital or hospice transfer, forgetting that such
a family will continue to behave in the same manner wherever the patient
is. The patient's welfare is certainly important but so also are the health
and happiness of the other carers, and particularly the spouse or partner
of the patient. What can the doctor and nurse do in such an unhappy
situation?

One answer is to have a family conference. All family members are asked
to attend and its importance stressed. It is led by either the doctor or the
nurse but, if at all possible, they should both be present. For the sake of
description here we shall assume the doctor is chairing it. He thanks people
for coming, sets a time limit (usually between 30 and 60 minutes), and
then explains how the meeting will be conducted. He opens by saying he
and nurse take it for granted that everyone present wants what is best for
John (as we shall call him here). Everyone has questions they want to ask
about him and his care, and problems and issues they want to raise, some
in relation to other family members. Everyone is sad, some are feeling
helpless, and it is assumed everyone wants to help other family members.
He emphasizes that everyone will get a chance to speak but no one is to
speak until it is their turn to do so.

The doctor then explains everything about John—diagnosis, treatment
past and present, the care principles being followed, and the plans to keep
him at home as long as possible, etc. He then goes round the group asking
each person in turn if they have any questions for him or nurse. Each is
answered honestly and simply, no opportunity being given for discussion
or arguments between members, but only with the doctor or nurse.

The doctor then says everyone has their own fears, doubts about coping,
anger, even guilt, apprehensions about the future. Now is the time to
mention them, even if it hurts to do so, even if they involve other family
members. Again he looks to each person in turn. No one is allowed to
retaliate or verbally attack anyone else.

Finally, when a great deal of anger and frustration has been released he
asks what each person feels they can bring to the situation to help with

John's care. Each person has to offer something. At this point, perhaps surprisingly, someone will offer to sit by him at night, another feeling unable to do that will offer to do the shopping, another to look after the children, and so it goes on. Soon a roster has been devised, everyone has been surprised at others' sadness and sense of helplessness, and even disputes have quietened down. The meeting is brought to a close with the doctor thanking everyone and complimenting them on their caring and willingness to help each other. Just before the meeting breaks up he slips in that he and nurse obviously cannot be explaining things to each and every member of the family, so who volunteers to be the channel for communication, the person who will carry the questions and take back the answers? This makes communicating much easier for all concerned. The traumatically dysfunctional family is effective again.

If, for some reason, it is decided not to have a family conference it is still essential to have one member of the family designated as the intermediary between the professionals and the extended family. The professionals must make it clear that neither the doctor nor the nurse have time to spend in family arguments and mutual blame sessions. They also need to be told how upsetting it is for the patient to hear, or be conscious of, bickering and disagreements in the house.

Bringing it all together

Daunting as some of this may have sounded, it is not so. Much of it and how to handle it is common sense, always provided we remember that the patient and probably most of the carers have never gone though any of this before. They are novices and very aware of that.

They need guidance not lectures, understanding not platitudes. In a sense they need friends as much as they need doctors and nurses, although the ideal is when the doctor and nurse have become friends of the family, almost members of the family they are working to help.

Patients need to be assured that someone is looking after the family, although often they will ask few questions and expect no details. They can usually sense when their loved ones are being cared for. At the same time the family wants to be sure the patient is getting the best possible care, from the professionals and from themselves, and will then be glad of simple support and guidance for their own personal needs. When each knows that the others are cared for, all is well and tensions fall.

5

Spiritual and religious issues

It is increasingly being recognized that religion and spirituality are not the same thing. Having said that, neither is easy to define and many doctors and nurses feel that neither is their responsibility.

This brief chapter accepts that many are uncomfortable speaking about these subjects but it also recognizes that palliative care, or having a life-threatening illness, seems to bring them to the fore, making professional avoidance difficult. In fact, the authors believe that understanding some of the religious and spiritual issues faced by these patients is a core part of palliative care in the home.

Religious issues

Religion describes a faith, a philosophy in which we believe and which gives meaning to our life and how we live it. It is involves beliefs, doctrines, and dogmas, and practices deemed important to the development of our faith, such as prayer, the reading of sacred texts such as the Bible, sacraments, anointing, personal discipline. Some religions have strict dietary rules, others injunctions concerning clothing, alcohol, fasting, forms of worship, and so forth. Without exception, all religions are about a God or gods and our relationship with and responsibility to the god(s).

Traditionally in the West we have regarded a person's religion, their faith, as a very personal matter. Like sex and, until recently, salaries, it was considered ill-mannered to discuss it. What a person believed and how they practised their faith was a matter for them and them alone, not even for their trusted family doctors, unless they chose to speak to them of their faith. For that reason, and because most feel ill-equipped to discuss faith or to deal with issues and problems arising from it, doctors have studiously avoided it in their dealings with patients.

It is often said that we now live in an agnostic, 'post-Christian' society, one where religion has little place, where fewer and fewer people either profess a faith or attend any form of worship. Nevertheless, experience shows that the more seriously ill a person is, particularly with a life-threatening illness, the more they recall the religious teaching and beliefs of their youth and return to religion for comfort. Years of lapsed belief and observance give way to a willingness to see the priest or minister or teacher, even a willingness to take a sacrament or to be anointed.

How are members of the primary care team to handle this sensitive matter?

The first point to make is that they should be prepared to facilitate but never to proselytize. They should demonstrate to the patient that, as in all matters concerning his or her welfare, they are ready to listen and to assist when they are asked to and able to. In relation to religion, terminally ill people can be said to fall into four groups.

1. There are those with an active faith, whether or not they speak much about it. They are probably in touch with their religious adviser and fellow believers. The doctor needs do no more than acknowledge this and, as always in medical practice, respect the patient's beliefs and customs. The biggest problem arises when someone apparently loses their faith: it has always seemed adequate and now it fails them. Perhaps it had never been tested or was an immature faith but, for whatever reason, they now feel unsupported and ashamed. It should be noted that this can affect even those whose faith is expected to be strong, such as members of the clergy and other professionals in the church or religious organizations. It may require direct questioning by the doctor to elicit the problem, which is then best dealt with by someone, usually a clergyman, who has encountered the problem.

2. There are those who perhaps once had a faith or a connection with a church or religious community but have fallen away from it. The doctor's responsibility is to sound out the patient to ask if they feel it might help to reactivate that connection. This can be done quite simply and sensitively. 'At times like this people often say their faith helps them. Is that the way it is with you? Is there any way I can help you get in touch again in case it might help? If there is, you must not hesitate to say so.' The doctor might then be asked what he knows of the local priest or vicar, or spiritual leaders of other faiths, or how approachable they are.

3. There is a relatively small group who have thought everything through and remain not agnostic but atheist. They feel no need for religion in any form and will be able to say so to a doctor who raises the subject or offers to assist. Their wishes must be respected but the doctor must not be surprised if there is a change of mind as the illness progresses. Once again there can be embarrassment and the doctor needs to put the patient at ease. The relatives are likely to be as surprised as the patient that such a change can occur.

4. The final group, and probably the largest one in our society today, is made up of those who have never thought seriously about religion. Life may have been good to them, with no major crises or tragedies until this mortal illness, so they may never had felt a need for a god or a faith in any form. The family doctor can expect them to give it some thought and not be surprised when, using the introduction suggested above, they say they would like to meet someone who can speak to them about 'the things that matter' as they describe faith. 'My wife still goes to church, though I don't, so perhaps her vicar would be willing to come round.' All the doctor then needs to do is to show interest.

It is worth noting that relatives are often very embarrassed by issues of religion as they affect the patient. They are either certain their faith is adequate, or surprised and embarrassed if it appears to be shaky, or at a loss to know what to say or do if a previously agnostic relative brings up the subject. 'He's gone all religious, doctor.'

One of the delights of working in a primary care team is that over the years you come to know many of the patients and families very well indeed and become accepted as a friend as much as their doctor. Touching on matters of faith becomes infinitely easier than it would when working in a hospital. Sometimes a patient will know of the doctor's faith or religion, or at least feel free to mention it. Whilst not an opportunity to promote one's own faith or impose it on others, it is nevertheless an opportunity for the doctor or nurse to say how it helps them, and in so doing removing any embarrassment or reticence the patient feels.

The clergy and leaders of other faiths, many of whom are much better trained in listening to and helping the dying than the medical profession, often say they find it helpful to have clinical information about the patient. By this they mean some idea of the prognosis ('are we talking about days, weeks, or months, doctor?'), what treatment is being given ('it helps to know if they are to have surgery or chemotherapy'), what the person has been told, and, equally important, what the nearest and dearest have been told.

It goes without saying that much as the doctor and nurse appreciate how helpful the information might be, they cannot disclose any part of it without the explicit consent of the patient. When asked if such things can be discussed with the clergyman, most patients agree when reassured it will go no further.

One final point about religion and faith, said with much respect for those whose faith means everything to them. As patients get near the end of life they are sometimes not as helped as you might expect them to be by absolute certainty. Some religious people seem to entertain no doubts whatsoever. They mean well but their total conviction can inadvertently upset those whose faith is currently being sorely tried. For that reason it is not uncommon for a dying person to ask not to be visited by a chaplain or priest, preferring a layperson.

Caring for someone of a different faith, or from a different ethnic background, can be exceedingly challenging. It is so easy inadvertently to say the wrong thing or do the wrong thing, leaving people upset or even angry at one of the saddest times in their lives.

Spiritual issues

Spirituality is usually said to be the search for existential meaning. It is the questions and the mysteries and the anomalies Man must have expressed since time began, and presumably will continue to articulate forever.

Why must Man suffer and eventually die? Why do some die so young? Why does Man suffer so much? What is the meaning of life? Life feels so unfair! Why do the good die young and some wicked people enjoy a life of health? Is there a God? Does having a faith make any difference? Does it matter whether or not we lead a 'good' life? What have I to show for my life? I feel undervalued. The list is endless.

It might be assumed that a person with a strong religious faith will have no such problems, his faith making sense of everything that happens in his life and the world around him. For the fortunate few this is true. For most people, however, faith does not guarantee peace of mind or freedom from existential questions. They seem to affect and afflict most people. Paradoxically, the better the palliative care being offered, the more relaxed the patient becomes with his or her professional carers, the more such questions and doubts they express. It is as if freeing them from pain and helping them to speak freely of whatever troubles them liberates them. Within a week or two most patients seem to enjoy ventilating their spiritual problems. The unfortunate thing is that they seem to expect answers. There are none!

Once again, how should the family doctor or community nurse respond?

It is important to remember several things which may not, at first, be self-evident.

- Patients enjoy and benefit from ventilating feelings but do not necessarily expect answers. They do, however, need to be invited to speak of such things.

- Although some spiritual questions sound religious, they are not; but, as we have implied, a strong faith might have many of the answers or explanations.

- Every person's death is unique to them but, to a point, they are relieved to know others have experienced something similar to them.

- Many people go through life without giving deep thoughts to things and are disturbed when they find themselves asking existential questions. Sometimes the intensity of their feelings surprises or alarms them.

- Most people only ask difficult questions or raise profound issues when they have no other anguishes to occupy their thoughts. Palliative care must be effective before spiritual issues raise their heads.

The presence of spiritual problems may be suspected, even when the patient does not report them, when depression features without the cardinal features of low self-esteem, altered sleep pattern, and poor concentration.

The vast majority of patients receiving palliative care are helped by learning that others have asked, and still ask, the same questions. They are helped when they hear that 'even the doctor' has thought the same thoughts and asked the same questions. Sometimes, simply replying 'Oh, I wish I had the answer to that. I have asked myself that question more times than I can remember' seems to help people.

Everyone wants to feel needed and valued. The nearer we get to the end of life the more this is so. Excellent palliative care does not necessarily help a dying person to feel either needed or valued. It can make them more distressed. People are doing everything possible to befriend them and make them comfortable but, they ask, are they useful in any way, are they needed for anything now that they have such a short time to live? This is one of the greatest challenges of palliative care—how to show someone they are still needed, still useful, and still valued. Smothering them with kindness is not the answer.

They have to be helped to see how their children and grandchildren value them and still learn from them, how their quiet example is an inspiration to others, how even the doctor and nurses learn from their lives.

What seems not to help is to launch into some philosophical discourse or soul-searching exercise. Like it or not, Man has asked these questions since he began recording his thoughts and his teachings. If we are still asking them, there can be no simple answers. In many ways it seems to be like therapeutics; if one drug always worked we would not be using so many, all claiming to do so!

It is always helpful, as with every other aspect of palliative care in the home, to record that the patient raised any of these issues and ask about them on a subsequent visit. 'Did you ever get in touch with that minister you were talking about, by the way?' or 'After I left you yesterday I thought a lot about what you had been telling me. I hope it helped you because it certainly set me thinking.'

Finally, whether dealing with religious or spiritual issues, it is worth remembering that there are few things less helpful and more upsetting for the terminally ill person and the grieving relatives than platitudes. No matter how well-intentioned, they never help. Constructive silence is infinitely preferable.

6

Emergencies in palliative care

Palliative care, like other branches of medicine, should be proactive rather than reactive, anticipating problems and taking the necessary action to prevent them if possible. Sometimes this is not possible and crises develop, presenting the primary care team with genuine emergencies. As with any medical emergency, failure to act speedily and appropriately may lead to tragedy and disaster. Furthermore, it can leave the relatives with even sadder memories, often coloured by anger and surprise that the doctor could let the patient down at this critical time in the care. It is a sad fact that when bereaved relatives look back on the care their loved one received they seem to overlook the weeks or months of excellent care and home visiting. What they recall vividly was the emergency and what they perceive as the doctor's or nurse's lack of skill in handling it. This chapter details the most common emergencies encountered when providing palliative care in the home.

Spinal cord compression (SCC)

This is a complication of malignant disease, usually of breast, bronchus, prostate, cervix, and thyroid. Any patient known to have spinal metastases of any of these primaries should be regarded as being at risk of this complication, particularly if the metastases are in the mid and lower dorsal spine.

There may be no warning symptoms, but usually careful questioning reveals some problem in voiding urine—hesitancy, a poor stream, or retention with overflow.

The only other warning sign is slight weakness or numbness in one or both legs. The patient may describe this as unsteadiness and both patient and carers understandably put it down to his general frailty. The tragedy is when the doctor does the same.

Paralysis, developing very suddenly with no accompanying pain, is most likely due to a vascular accident but nevertheless the doctor should manage the case as he would if metastatic compression was suspected. It is important to remember that pain is not a consistent warning feature.

The emergency itself may present with intense bilateral nerve root pain radiating from the affected area but more usually it is silent, painless. The first sign that there is a crisis is when the patient develops urinary retention, accompanied by weakness or paralysis of the legs, dysaesthesia or total anaesthesia with diminution or loss of reflexes and inability to stand or walk. Examination confirms these neurological features and may also demonstrate hypoaesthesia below the affected dermatome—a sensory level.

Management

Emergency decompression is called for. It may be by surgery, by radiotherapy or by steroids. No time can be wasted.

+ If diagnosed within 24 hours of it happening, neurosurgical decompression may be effective. To ensure that appropriate treatment is received as speedily as possible the doctor should phone the nearest neurosurgical centre and discuss the case with the surgeon on call. The patient will have magnetic resonance imaging (MRI) rather than a myelogram before surgery. The surgeon may decline to operate if the patient has a very short prognosis (as with some bronchogenic carcinomas) or if the extent of the spinal secondaries is such that operation may lead to further spinal collapse.

+ If the compression is over 24 hours old, or if the neurosurgeon recommends such a course, the patient may be better treated with radiotherapy. Once again this is an emergency and must be discussed on the telephone with the radiotherapist rather than sending the patient to an Accident and Emergency Department with the inevitable delays.

+ When neither option is available, high-dose dexamethasone occasionally helps and will be given by the family doctor in the home. In the United Kingdom the starting dose is 24 milligrams in the first 24 hours, preferably given either intravenously or by an intramuscular injection, followed by 20 milligrams, 16 milligrams, 12 milligrams, and 8 milligrams, all given orally, on succeeding days. Any benefit will be obvious within 48 hours, often within 24 hours. If no benefit whatsoever is demonstrable within 5 days, the drug should be discontinued. It should be remembered that dexamethasone also acts as a cerebral stimulant when given in the second half of the day. The patient and relatives need to be warned that sleep may be disturbed.

◆ Even when the SSC is handled as an emergency, several hours may elapse between the doctor being called and the patient finally being admitted for whatever mode of decompression is chosen. If there is any possibility that in that interval the patient will develop urinary retention, it is a kindness to catheterize before leaving home.

If the SCC was discovered late or the treatment fails, the new challenge is how and where to care for the paraplegic, but probably pain-free, patient. The decision will partly depend on the facilities of the home, the availability of nurses, and the ability and availability of relatives. The mean survival time of an otherwise relatively well cancer patient who becomes paraplegic is 3 months, a long time for a family to care for someone so dependent, but probably shorter than most imagine.

Superior vena caval obstruction (SVCO)

This is a complication of mediastinal adenopathy, itself a common feature of the lymphomas, bronchogenic carcinoma, breast and thyroid carcinoma. For that reason it should be remembered and looked for in such patients. Unlike SCC it develops relatively slowly and insidiously, often over a week or two, rather than dramatically.

The patient reports worsening dyspnoea at rest, and at night when it might mimic paroxysmal nocturnal dypnoea.

The signs are dramatic and pathognomonic. Collateral veins appear on the upper half of the anterior chest wall, oedematous bags show under the eyes, the jugular venous pressure (JVP) is raised, and, in the advanced stages, the patient becomes cyanosed. The patient appears puffed out and bloated as if holding his breath or straining.

Management

The diagnosis must be established and then treated appropriately. This is a condition where discussion with a specialist in palliative medicine or oncology can prove very useful. The aim is to reduce the adenopathy and so relieve the obstruction on the SVC.

1. If the patient has not already had full-dose radiotherapy to the mediastinum, this should be organized with the radiotherapist as a matter of urgency.

LIVERPOOL
JOHN MOORES UNIVERSITY
AVRIL ROBARTS LRC
TITHEBARN STREET
LIVERPOOL L2 2ER
TEL. 0151 231 4022

2. If radiotherapy is not feasible, for whatever reason, the patient should be treated at home with dexamethasone. The dosing regimen is exactly as for SCC.

Benefit should be obvious within 48 hours, often within 24 hours. Dexamethasone is continued, 2–4 milligrams each morning, as maintenance therapy indefinitely. The prognosis is that of the underlying malignancy. If treatment is not given or is unsuccessful, plans must be made to care for an increasingly frightened, very dyspnoeic patient.

Convulsions

Here we are dealing with convulsions occurring for the first time in patients already diagnosed as having an advanced disease, not as the presenting features.

Convulsions occur in 10 per cent of terminally ill patients, usually as a result of cerebral secondaries most commonly from primaries in bronchus or breast, and in melanoma. It is important to remember that before the first fit their presence may not have been suspected or diagnosed even on a brain scan. Less commonly, the fits are a result of neurosurgery or cerebrovascular accident (CVA).

An important question is whether or not the patient and/or the relatives should be warned that convulsions may occur. There can be no dogmatic advice on this. Many would argue that to warn the patient, already burdened with the diagnosis and failing health, is only adding to that burden and increasing his apprehensions.

That seems wise counsel, but may not be true for the relatives. Seeing a person having a fit for the first time is alarming for anyone, but probably more so when the relative was not expecting it, had no idea what to do, and probably suspected that it heralded an imminent death. The last thing that the patient needs, and the primary care team wants, is an emergency admission to hospital (quite possibly not the one known to the patient). Their ability to care for the patient at home will largely depend on the relatives' ability to care for the patient there, itself contingent on them understanding what is happening and what they can do to help. On balance it is better to advice the relatives when there is a strong likelihood of the patient having a fit. Time spent explaining what happens and what to do, in as relaxed a manner as possible, is time well spent in palliative care.

Management

1. If the doctor can be on the scene within minutes the patient should be given intravenous diazepam 10 milligrams at the rate of 1 milligram per minute. An alternative is intravenous midazolam 5–10 milligrams at the same rate. Perhaps it does not need to be said that diazepam should not be given intramuscularly because it takes more than an hour to achieve adequate plasma levels, and that midazolam produces total amnesia for the time around the event.

2. When such a rapid response by the doctor is impossible, the relatives should be left with a supply of, and instructions how to use, rectal diazepam solution (not suppository). The dose is 20 milligrams for an adult, expected to be effective for 3 hours.

3. Just as the relatives need to be instructed in giving the rectal solution, they also need to be taught to remove dentures, loosen clothing, and maintain an airway.

4. After the first convulsion the patient should be put on to maintenance anticonvulsants such as phenytoin, 300 milligrams nightly, or midazolam 30 milligrams over 24 hours added to the medication in the syringe driver if that is in use.

5. The question arises what the doctor should do if papilloedema is found when the patient is examined after the fit. Presumably there is raised intracranial pressure. Should the patient be put on to dexamethasone or the dose be increased if already on it?

6. If the patient has advanced malignancy it can be assumed that there are cerebral secondaries. Whether or not the patient should have a brain scan depends on the general condition of the patient, the possible time delay in getting it done and getting the results, and the problems of transporting a frail patient. The only benefit of such a scan is to confirm the presence of secondaries and whether they might benefit from hemi-brain irradiation or, less commonly, surgical excision of a solitary lesion. Whatever the scan findings the patient should be put on to dexamethasone to reduce cerebral oedema. The starting oral dose is 16 milligrams per day, reducing every second day by 2 milligrams to a maintenance dose of 2–4 milligrams per day, all doses taken before mid-afternoon.

7. In the patient already on dexamethasone when the fit occurred, the dose should be increased to 8 milligrams and maintained there for 4 days before reducing it as just described. It has to be anticipated that

each time this boosted dose regimen is used, the benefits will be less and less dramatic. The time will come, and the relatives need to be warned in advance of it, that giving high-dose steroids will not help.

This is an appropriate place to remind readers that the steroids, including dexamethasone, have many more adverse effects than dyspepsia, gastrointestinal bleeding, and weight gain with Cushingoid features (see p. 48).

Haemorrhage

Contrary to what most laypeople and even some professionals may think, catastrophic haemorrhage is rare in the terminally ill. Most family doctors and community nurses will go through their whole professional lives without seeing a case. This, however, is not likely to reassure anyone concerned.

Haemorrhage is likely to be from the upper gastrointestinal tract or the chest when a malignancy has eroded into a major vessel. Less likely is a massive haemoptysis from tuberculosis, although the resurgence of this disease makes it possible.

Less dramatic bleeding is common but does not constitute an emergency. It should be expected from the bladder in patients with bladder, prostatic, or cervical carcinoma; from the vagina in uterine and cervical carcinoma; from the mouth in patients with pharyngeal, laryngeal, and tonsillar carcinoma; as haematemesis in patients with gastric carcinoma or as a result of taking non-steroidal anti-inflammatory drugs (NSAIDs) with steroids.

Although the lesser haemorrhages are not truly medical emergencies, they are alarming for the patient and the relatives who suspect that there might be a massive bleed or that they signify impending death. Reassurance is not easy and requires considerable skill if urgent and possibly unnecessary admission to hospital is to be avoided.

Management

1. When there is a massive haemorrhage the aim of any intervention is to sedate the patient as speedily as possible. Once again the two best drugs are intravenous diazepam given as 1 milligram per minute up to 10 milligrams or intravenous midazolam given at the same rate up to 5–10 milligrams. If the patient is already on one of these drugs the dose given intravenously should be one-sixth of the total daily dose. Opioids are not indicated for sedation.

2. Whether or not the patient should be admitted to hospital once adequate sedation has been achieved depends on the usual factors—what might be achieved by admission, the hazards of the journey, the wishes of the patient, the wishes and the coping ability of the relatives, amongst others. The judgement is a fine one. It has always to be borne in mind that, unless specifically requested not to do so, the admitting doctor may embark on heroic measures totally inappropriate for a patient in the final stage of life, something that most terminally ill people do not want. Even telephoning the hospital in advance may not prevent this happening. The doctor, in consultation with the community nurse if that is possible, will also want to gauge whether or not the family will cope, what assistance they will need, what different medication might be useful, whether night nurses should be brought in, and what additional information and advice they need if the patient stays at home.

Finally it should be borne in mind that if an ambulance is summoned to the house and the patient has just died or is about to die, the paramedics are not permitted to use their discretion whether or not to resuscitate and then take the patient to the nearest hospital They must do so unless written instructions to the contrary have been left in the house by the family doctor. This can be very distressing for relatives.

Acute hypercalcaemia

Most usually, hypercalcaemia develops over weeks or days. Seldom does it present as an emergency, but when it does it can be as dramatic as its response to appropriate treatment. The features and treatment of hypercalcaemia presenting slowly are discussed elsewhere in this book.

Even in an emergency it usually becomes clear that the patient has had features suggestive of hypercalcemia for several days—increasing thirst, polyuria, weakness and tiredness, and even modest confusion—all attributed to the underlying illness. The confusional state gets much worse suddenly, often with features of paranoia and aggression, the whole demeanour of the patient becoming different from normal.

Although these features strongly suggest hypercalcaemia, the diagnosis can only be confirmed by biochemical measurements of calcium and albumin. The priority in the home is to sedate the patient as described under haemorrhage, although smaller doses will be needed, before taking off blood for urgent testing.

Subsequent management depends on the biochemistry. Unless the calcium is only minimally elevated (unlikely if the picture was that of an emergency), in which case the patient can remain at home, admission to hospital for a few days will be needed.

Once again, as is so often the case with emergencies in palliative care in the home, a key question is whether much will be gained by hospital admission. If, prior to the features of hypercalcaemia in the previous few days, the patient was reasonably well and enjoying a good quality of life, then correction of the hypercalcaemia must be regarded as medically and ethically essential. Within 48–72 hours the patient may be home again and be maintained normocalcaemic for weeks or even a few months. If, on the other hand, the hypercalcaemic crisis was but another sign of dramatic decline within a short space of time, correction of the biochemical imbalance will not improve the quality of life and arrangements should be made for continuing care at home. If this is the course of action decided upon, the relatives will need to be told why, and be warned that confusion will be a feature of the final week or so of life.

Acute urinary retention

Although seldom presenting as an emergency, acute urinary retention is a common crisis in palliative care, calling for urgent attention. In this group of patients the causes are:

◆ tricyclic antidepressants

◆ opioids

◆ faecal impaction in the rectum

◆ clot retention

◆ spinal cord compression

◆ urinary tract infection

◆ benign prostatic hyperplasia.

The management is immediate catheterization before attempting to deal with whatever underlying problem is identified. Although urologists would understandably advise self-catheterization rather than leaving in an indwelling catheter, most palliative medicine physicians would use the latter if the problem was deemed irreversible, suggesting to the community nurse that it be lavaged weekly with normal saline.

Pathological fractures

The fragility of bones in the elderly and frail is well known even if they do not have metastases. Immobilization of the elderly, for whatever reason, leads rapidly to decalcification. Fractures can occur with minimal trauma, even during nursing and handling procedures. A pathological fracture should always be suspected when a patient with cancer reports a new bone/joint pain anywhere in the body. A thorough examination is essential.

Often the site is obvious, as in the clavicle or surgical neck of humerus. In other sites it may be missed, in spite of the intense pain being reported by the patient, often because a thorough examination is not carried out. Some patients are admitted to a specialist palliative care unit or hospice because of 'uncontrollable pain', only to be found to have a surgically correctable fracture of the femoral neck. This is a timely reminder that, when providing palliative care in the home, every new pain, and every old pain which has suddenly got worse, demands thorough investigation before adjusting the analgesia.

Management

Unless the patient is in extremis, admission to an appropriate unit is essential. The only possible exceptions are:

1. Fractured clavicle can and should be treated at home unless the fracture is thought to be pathological and it is thought desirable to have the metastasis irradiated.

2. Fractured ribs can be made very comfortable with local anaesthetic infiltrated into the site, or preferably an intercostal block for which a palliative medicine physician might be invited in. Strapping is contraindicated.

Fractured neck of femur should be operated on unless the prognosis for the patient is deemed to be no more than days. Prior to sending the patient to hospital, 10 millilitres of 2 per cent lignocaine can be injected around the fracture site to make the ambulance journey less uncomfortable.

If it is decided to keep the patient at home because it is thought that the prognosis is a matter of days, the site can be bathed in lignocaine infused via a fine bore polythene cannula connected to a syringe driver, using no more than 20 millilitres per day. Rotation of the affected leg can be prevented with sandbags placed either side of it.

Acute intestinal obstruction

This is a common problem, although, usually, after the initial episode which may be the presenting feature of the underlying malignancy, it is subacute. It is often recurrent, as in the case of women with ovarian carcinoma, when close on 50 per cent develop it. Here, therefore, we are looking at an event likely to be encountered many times in family practice, but different from the first attack which led to the diagnosis of intra-abdominal malignancy.

This distinction is important. In the undiagnosed patient the management will always include 'drip and suction' and usually laparotomy. In the recurrent attacks of subacute intestinal obstruction that the patient may subsequently suffer, 'drip and suction' are not mandatory. In fact, hospital admission is not mandatory.

The clinical features differ from those of the first attack. There may be pain of a colicky nature but it is rarely as severe as in the initial attack and may not be a major feature at all. Because it is usually a partial obstruction, the patient may pass a little flatus but usually no faeces. The key issue is whether there is vomiting and how soon it occurs after a small drink. If the patient vomits almost immediately, the obstruction is high, around the pylorus or upper small intestine. If the patient seldom vomits but has increasing abdominal distension and a tympanitic abdomen, the obstruction is in the lower small bowel or the colon. Finally it has to be remembered that there might be multiple sites of obstruction, particularly in ovarian carcinoma and when the patient has been subjected to several abdominal operations, resulting in adhesions.

Management

1. The first thing the family doctor has to ask is whether the obstruction is likely to be at a single site or multiple sites. The former may be amenable to surgical management and therefore calls for admission to hospital, the latter will not and might be managed at home.

2. The second question is whether or not the patient needs 'drip and suction'. High obstructions lead to such recurrent vomiting and inability to keep any fluids down that 'drip and suction' is needed. Lower obstructions can safely be managed without 'drip and suction' if oral hydration is skilfully managed and colic controlled with antispasmodics. It is quite possible to manage lower obstructions at home.

3. The best analgesic is hyoscine butylbromide, given as intermittent 6 hourly injections of 20 milligrams or 120 milligrams over 24 hours via syringe driver, usefully combined with an opioid.

After dealing with the emergency, the doctor and nurse will have to consider dietary advice for the patient, the possible use of docusate as an osmotic faecal softener, and whether or not octreotide, a somatostatin analogue, is called for. These are discussed elsewhere in this book.

The doctor should never hesitate to contact a palliative medicine specialist to discuss such patients.

Acute panic attacks

As discussed elsewhere in this book, anxiety and apprehension are very common features in patients under palliative care. Inevitably, there are occasions when the anxiety builds up to a crescendo, a panic attack, and it is that we are referring to here.

The borderline between severe anxiety and panic is impossible to define, but whereas frightening anxiety might respond to reassurance, an opportunity to 'talk it through', and a mild short-acting anxiolytic, the person suffering panic attack can scarcely speak, does not listen, cannot sit still, and is physically and emotionally distressed. No amount of reassuring or sympathetic companionship helps.

Here we shall deal only with the acute attack and its management. As soon as possible after it has settled, the members of the primary care team must plan future care. They should ask such questions as who will explore the patient's fears, they should answer his questions, explain all that needs to be explained, help the relatives, and decide what medication (if any) might help to prevent future attacks.

Management

In a severe panic attack the priority is sedation of the patient, not leisurely talking through of problems and fears.

1. The best drug is subcutaneous midazolam 5–10 milligrams given as a bolus, and expected to show an effect within 3–5 minutes and last for 3 hours. It is amnesogenic, so the doctor and carers need to remember that afterwards the patient may have no memory whatsoever of the incident or what was said. Rarely the drug may need to be given intravenously, at a rate not exceeding 1 milligram a minute. If the patient has been on long-term benzodiazepines, or is currently on them as

part of the palliative care regimen, the dose suggested above should be doubled.

2. A less acceptable alternative is intravenous diazepam 5–10 milligrams, given at a rate of 1 milligram a minute. Because of the long half-life of this drug and its metabolites, sedation may persist for days.

Certain things do not help. They include increasing the opioids, chlorpromazine or any of the phenothiazines, and even haloperidol, useful as it is on a long-term basis. It cannot be stressed strongly enough that panic attacks must be energetically treated if the relatives are to be reassured about what they are doing and if the patient is to remain at home.

7

Ethical issues

Ethical issues arise at all stages of a patient's care and are an integral part of medical and nursing decision making. Ethical dilemmas have no easy solution but doctors and nurses can encourage patients and their families to express their views and to become involved in taking decisions. Good communication skills facilitate the formation of a partnership between patients and professionals. In the context of such a partnership, both parties become more informed of each other's view and thus can work together to achieve the best outcome for the patient. This chapter will focus on ethical issues encountered by primary care teams providing palliative care at home.

Communication

If patients are to be in a position to be involved in decisions about their care and to plan for the future, they need honest information about the diagnosis, prognosis, treatment options, side-effects, and sources of professional support. Thus, good communication is an essential part of an ethical approach to patient care. Good communication helps to maintain a trusting relationship between professional and patient. Uncertainties exist for both patients and their carers, but these may be reduced if they are confronted and discussed. Advances in medical technology have raised patient's expectations; consequently, part of the professional's duty is to encourage patients to have realistic hopes and allow them time to adjust to their changing circumstances.

The most common reason for complaints against family doctors is poor communication. It is not just what we do that matters to patients and relatives, but the manner in which we do it. Patients are often anxious and therefore less able to take in new information. They may misinterpret words, such as 'response' for cure, or they may assume that treatments such as palliative chemotherapy or radiotherapy are directed towards a cure rather than symptom control. Patients, like all of us, are inconsistent; they may block information. A patient may ask his general practitioner what was found at operation. The doctor has a letter in his notes from the surgeon, stating that the patient understands that the cancer was not fully resected and appreciates the poor prognosis. The experienced family doctor will understand the reason for this apparent paradox, that the patient was in denial, and gently explore the patient's understanding of his condition and explain the findings at the patient's pace. It is never helpful to patients to be critical of colleagues. It is impossible for the many professionals caring for a patient to speak with one voice, so that patient and relatives all hear and understand the same thing. Indeed, nurses spend a great deal of time explaining to patients what the doctor has said to them.

Communication between professionals takes a great deal of time, but it is time well spent. One of the prime ethical duties is to respect the patient as an autonomous individual. One powerful mechanism for ensuring this respect is a requirement for obtaining informed consent from a patient before embarking on a medical intervention.

Informed consent

All medical interventions carry the potential for threatening a patient's autonomy. Patients with advanced disease can appear physically frail and are vulnerable to well-intentioned but possibly unwanted medical interventions. Doctors are experts on the medical aspects of the patient. However, they are not experts in the social, spiritual, or emotional aspects of the patient's life. These non-medical issues might be of much greater significance to the patient than the medical concerns. The doctor needs to beware of the urge to do good, which drives paternalism, and to ensure he/she listens to the patient as an 'expert' in his or her own right. A requirement for informed consent ensures a sharing of power and knowledge between doctor and patient. Patient consent acts as a mechanism to protect autonomy against paternalistic interventions.

Informed consent is thus much more than the signing of a piece of paper before an operation, but is a dynamic process where professionals and patients form a partnership. Within this relationship, both become more aware of each other's needs and can work together to achieve the best possible outcome for the patient.

Confidentiality

A health care professional has a duty not to divulge information about a patient to a third party without the explicit consent of the patient. Without a requirement for confidentiality it would be impossible to build a trusting relationship with the patient. However, as we have discussed earlier in this book, palliative care demands a team approach if we are to treat the whole person, addressing psychological, spiritual, and social concerns, as well as the physical ones. If teamwork is to be effective, then information about the patient needs to be shared amongst members of the team. How is this to be done whilst still retaining trust? One solution is to explain from the outset that you are a member of a team and to ask the patient's permission to share this information with the team. In addition, one can use the 'need to know' guide. In other words, there are different levels of information which can be shared with other professionals who need this information in order to help the patient. If there is doubt in a professional's mind, it is always best to clarify with the patient whether he/she is content to share the information with another professional.

Sharing information amongst professionals bound by ethical codes of confidentiality is generally accepted and rarely gives rise to ethical problems. Much more difficult is the question of how much information should be divulged to relatives and other carers who often demand that rules of confidentiality be broken. They have the best of motives, to protect the patient from the bad news. Patients are usually fully aware of their diagnosis and may ironically also try to protect relatives by putting on a brave face. It is all too easy for the doctor and nurse to get drawn into this collusion, which only serves to isolate the patient. Open, honest communication with the patient and family together, from the beginning, will prevent collusion. If collusion exists, then the doctor and nurse need to explore with the relatives their reasons for withholding information, the emotional costs of deception, the likelihood of the patient being aware anyway, and the reasons why the patient would be better off having the information. The challenge for the family doctor is to negotiate permission from the relatives so that they feel involved in the patient's care. An insistence that it is the patient's right to know may be ethically correct but may serve to estrange the co-operation of those most involved in palliative care—the relatives.

Family doctors and community nurses need to meet so that each knows what has been said, what the relatives have asked and been told, and each must trust and respect the judgements and actions of fellow professionals working in the team.

Compassion

Compassion involves both a passive component of the capacity to feel with others and an active response to these feelings. Professionals who deny emotions and feelings of vulnerability in themselves and in their patients distance themselves from patients. Ethics is not simply a matter of rigid codes of behaviour but involves these emotional aspects of care, which are an integral part of the trusting relationship between professional and patient. Patients do not want pity but they do need doctors and nurses whom they can trust not to abandon them when active treatments are no longer appropriate.

Withdrawal of feeding and fluids

The aim of palliative care is the comfort of the patient. In deciding whether to withdraw feeding and fluids from patients dying of advanced disease, the doctor must consider the views of the patient and family. Relatives may feel a basic instinct to give fluids and nutrition to their loved one. They may perceive that he/she is dying from starvation or dehydration, rather than from their advanced disease, when they can no longer swallow solids or liquids. Nutritional support in the form of nasogastric tube feeding, a feeding gastrostomy, or even parenteral nutrition (TPN) may be appropriate at an earlier stage of the disease or to support a patient through radiotherapy or chemotherapy, which will shrink the tumour. At the end of life such measures may do little to make the patient more comfortable and may make some symptoms worse.

It must be emphasized that each case must be looked at individually; there can be no hard and fast rules. Doctors have a duty not to hasten death but also not to prolong suffering.

Time needs to be spent with relatives explaining that there is a difference between dying from dehydration and dehydration in patients dying from their cancer. Similarly, cancer cachexia is the result of metabolic changes that are different from those that occur in starvation. Intravenous fluids necessitate hospital admission and may do little to improve quality of life if the patient does not feel thirsty. The setting up of infusions gives a mixed message to relatives who may feel that this form of treatment is prolonging suffering in the dying patient. Intravenous infusions may also worsen some symptoms such as vomiting, incontinence, and respiratory secretions.

On the other hand, if the relatives have strong views that the patient would be better off with fluids, then doctors need to listen to this view, particularly if the patient is unable to make a decision. The legality of withdrawing hydration and feeding in the terminally ill has not been tested in the courts in Britain.

Decision making about withdrawal of fluids and nutrition is often difficult. It is one area where discussion between family doctors and specialist staff is advisable. If there are differences of professional view then these need to be debated and a consensus achieved. It is most disturbing for relatives if team members are giving different advice and opinions.

Advance directives or living wills

Some patients have made written directives known as living wills or advance directives, which state the conditions under which they would not wish to be resuscitated. They have arisen as a result of a fear of the inappropriate use of medical technology to keep people alive at all costs and irrespective of the patient's likely future quality of life, and because people do not wish to be a burden to their relatives.

General practitioners are in the best position to talk through these issues with the patient and family. The family doctor can reassure the patient that everything will be done to ease suffering and preserve dignity. Where the patient has made an advance directive, the general practitioner should inform hospital colleagues when the patient is admitted to hospital. Living wills have a legal force in Britain and should be respected by doctors. However, they are not legal unless they have described the precise clinical situation in advance. An advance directive cannot force a doctor to carry out a treatment that is inappropriate or futile.

Advance directives are not a substitute for honest communication between a patient and their doctor. Patients need to be reassured that they will have access to palliative care that does not prolong suffering but rather respects dignity and achieves good symptom control.

Euthanasia

Confusing definitions complicate the debate concerning euthanasia. Here we are not discussing a comfortable death with dignity but the deliberate ending of a patient's life at their request. Paradoxically, both sides of the euthanasia debate aim to relieve suffering; the pro-euthanasia lobby by intentionally ending life, and palliative care by meticulous symptom control and attention to psychological, spiritual, and social distress.

Physician-assisted suicide involves a doctor intentionally giving the patient advice or the means to commit suicide. Assisting a person to commit suicide is against the law in England, Wales, and Northern Ireland.

The detailed arguments surrounding euthanasia are beyond the scope of this small book. Those involved in palliative care need to be able to listen to the concerns of relatives who may find the prolonged dying of their loved one intolerable and demand that 'something must be done'. Sometimes the relatives may perceive the patient to be suffering and vocalize their distress, as 'I would not let a dog suffer like this'. These concerns require acknowledgement and a gentle exploration of the patient's or relatives view. Sometimes the fact that euthanasia is prohibited may be a help to the doctor who may respond by saying 'I understand what you are asking me to do, but I cannot deliberately shorten life, so let's look at what I can help with', or the doctor may reassure a patient that whilst she cannot shorten life, nor is she going to prolong suffering. The patient needs to have confidence that there are effective drugs to relieve physical suffering.

Some patients seem to fear a prolonged dying, sustained by an insensitive medical technology. Often a discussion about the principles of good palliative care reassures patients and relatives that the dying can be dignified and not involve physical suffering. The family doctor is in a unique position to anticipate these fears and to initiate an open, honest discussion with the patient and the family.

The euthanasia debate has nothing to do with the appropriate use of opioids in palliative care. The titration of opioids to relieve pain does not shorten life. The use of analgesics to relieve pain in the terminal phase is part of good medicine and nursing. The intention of the doctor or nurse to relieve a particular symptom is morally relevant to the debate. One of the sad consequences of the recent publicity in this area is that some doctors may fear to give appropriate analgesia in case they are criticized later by the media.

In dealing with these ethical dilemmas it is helpful to discuss the issues with colleagues, to document the reasons for giving drugs, and to keep good notes.

Dilemmas, by definition, have no easy answers. However, in the struggle to achieve the best outcome, we define the essence of good clinical practice.

8

Communication issues

It is often said that communications lie at the heart of good palliative care. If they are bad, it scarcely matters how good is the pain and symptom control. If they are good, it feels so much easier to help the patient. While all this is probably true, it can be said equally well about all clinical care and especially that in the patient's home. However, communication skills are every bit as important in hospital practice. Academic brilliance or technical wizardry seldom compensates for poor communication skills.

One problem is that most doctors and nurses know that they are good communicators but, sadly, those with whom they have to work are not! It is like car driving. If only others were as skilled and considerate drivers as we are, our roads would be safer and we would all get more pleasure out of our driving!

Many years spent as family doctors and consultants has brought this home to us. Family doctors often lament how inadequate are the letters they receive from consultants, detailing biochemical profiles and radiographic results but never mentioning what the patient has been told or how he reacted. When you speak to the consultant he says exactly the same about *his* family medicine colleague, *his* letters missing key information, not listing current medication, never mentioning admission to another hospital, and so on. Nurses often speak of how they have to interpret what doctors have said because the patient did not understand, while doctors criticize the nurses for the quality of their record keeping or for giving inaccurate information to patients, etc. None of us come out of this with many credit points.

What follows are suggestions only with regard to communications in palliative care. They are not intended as a treatise on communications in general. One basic principle simply must be stated, however, before looking at different situations—communications are as much about listening as about talking and telling. If we have not been trained, or trained ourselves, how to listen, then it hardly matters how well we pass on information to patients, relatives, and colleagues.

The sooner we stop thinking of communicating as passing on information the better. It is vastly more than that. It embraces listening, knowing when to speak and when to remain silent, how much to say and when to withhold some information, and how to modify how we do it according to the person with whom we are communicating.

Communications between doctor and patient

Perhaps this can be summarized to

- always be honest, difficult and painful as that may be
- demonstrate not only willingness to listen but skills in listening
- assure the patient that you will always give as much information and explanation as he/she wants at any one time
- always check how much the patient has taken in and understood of what has been said, no matter how simple was the message
- at each subsequent meeting or consultation on the same topic, check again what the patient remembered from the last meeting.

It is a myth that every patient wants to know everything about his condition. It is, however, true that every patient wants to be assured that whatever his doctor says is honest, is true. In palliative care, trust is important.

We are all tempted to dilute unpleasant facts to reduce the pain they produce. No matter how well-intentioned a reply or an explanation, if it was not honest it will later be seen by the patient as evidence that the doctor can be dishonest or less than truthful. People are usually happy for us to dilute the truth when they are the relatives trying to protect someone they love. It is another matter when they change roles and become the patient.

Here we must be totally honest and admit that many doctors dilute the truth, expressing important information in euphemistic terms, in a misguided effort to protect the patient. Every family doctor must remember times when they have had to undo some of the damage done. Some examples may help here.

The surgeon tells the patient he managed to 'get most of it away'. The doctor looks at a straight film and remarks 'no tumour to be seen on your X-ray'. The oncologist reads out a pathology report and interprets it to the patient as 'good news—no cancer cells in that gland we took out' but fails to say the cancer was known to have spread elsewhere. There is the doctor who keeps saying 'there is always something we can do' but does not manage to explain that there is no chemotherapy likely to be effective and the 'something' he mentioned is palliative care. Worse still, and unforgivable in our view, is the negative and defeatist 'palliative care is all we can offer, I'm afraid.'

The amount of information a patient wants, or feels he needs, varies from day to day. The macho man who boasts that he can take everything the doctor tells him soon asks for painful truths and information to be given to him in smaller morsels. The critical thing, in every conversation with the patient, is to ask how much they want to hear that day and to invite them to set the pace. After each morsel of information or explanation, pause and ask if the patient understands what you have said and if they would be kind enough to replay it back to you. Do the same again at the next meeting.

Self-evident as it may appear, what the patient may want to know may not be what the doctor or nurse feel is important, and vice versa. For that reason it helps to reassure the patient that you will explain as much as they want to hear but, first, would they mind explaining why they want to know something.

Some other points worth remembering in palliative care.

◆ Patients and relatives play games with each other and with their doctors. They say one thing to one and something different to another. They protect each other, and indeed themselves. A patient will claim he has never been told anything so that he does not have to speak about it to his relatives. Both parties convince themselves that they and they alone know 'the whole truth' and have managed to keep it from the other.

◆ Patients usually say different things to the different professionals caring for them. Hence the doctor will be told one thing, the nurse something else. For example, the palliative care patient will spontaneously report pain when the doctor visits, but when the nurse comes in may tell her that what worries him most is not the pain but the fact that his bowels have not moved for days. As research has demonstrated, patients tend to mention the things in which the different professionals seem to have been interested in the past. This is not 'playing one off against the other', but is a timely reminder that palliative care calls for a multiprofessional approach, if only to know everything which matters to the patient.

◆ Sometimes the word 'cancer' causes a complete system failure. Whatever the doctor says after that is not heard, no matter how positive or encouraging it is. If a euphemistic alternative is used, the patient and family should be left in no doubt that it is an alternative and should be told why you are doing so or you end up with the patient saying he is glad he just has a tumour and not a cancer.

♦ Patients hear what they want to hear, remember what is safe to remember, and delete a substantial amount of what we tell them. They know we cannot be precise about prognosis yet will take us literally when we try to answer their questions about prognosis. Some examples might illustrate this. 'I'm quite sure you are going to see Christmas and have a wonderful time with the family' is interpreted as dying between Christmas and New Year because 'if you had thought I'd see the New Year you would have said so, doctor!'

♦ Terminally ill people, as has been said thousands of times, are more concerned about the dying than the death—what will they have to suffer, will it be relieved, will the family be able to cope, will the family doctor be there and know what to do . . . ? Time need not be wasted chatting about death when it could better be spent relieving physical and emotional suffering, as this book outlines.

♦ As discussed much more fully in the chapter on symptom management, it is the significance to the patient of each symptom which matters, not its diagnostic significance to the doctor or nurse. This is critically important in all communications with the patient. The patient wants to know whether his dyspnoea will eventually asphyxiate him, not whether the doctor knows the diagnosis. The man with poorly relieved pain does not want platitudes and prayers so much as reassurance that it will not be pain that kills him. Always ask what lies at the back of the patient's question about a symptom. 'I can see you're really worried about being muddled last night. I'll explain it to you but first, tell me why it upset you so much. Am I right in thinking it's because your mother died in a psychiatric hospital?' The family doctor is often in a unique position to have that sort of information.

♦ All terminally ill people have spells of silence, no matter how loquacious they have been in the past. This has to be respected but it often helps to ask if they have 'something on their mind' they might find it helpful to share. On most occasions it turns out to be a spiritual issue, though they might not glorify it with such a description. Just knowing that the doctor or nurse understands is helpful to them.

♦ Palliative care patients are usually deeply concerned about their relatives and how they are coping. It is helpful for the doctor and nurse to demonstrate that they too are concerned for the relatives and are prepared to do all they can to help. All that is needed is the occasional observation such as 'Mary looks less tired today' or the opposite, 'Mary's looking tired, isn't she? Anything you would like me to do or to say which might help her?'

Having a mortal illness does not enhance either memory or intellectual acuity. There are two ways in which the patient may be helped to remember what was said. One is to record conversations and consultations on tape, as is now done in many hospital out-patient departments. The patient then takes the tape home to listen to and digest at leisure. They are encouraged to bring it back to the next session and ask whatever questions have arisen from it. The other thing to do, and found particularly useful in palliative care, is to encourage the patient and/or relatives to buy a little notebook. They carry it with them everywhere. At the front they write in what the doctor and nurse have said to them. At the back they list the questions or issues they want to mention to the doctor or nurse when next they meet. They are reminded that nothing is trivial. Whatever they want to ask or say is legitimate for the notebook.

The reader will have noticed that 'breaking bad news' has not been mentioned. That should have been done months or even years before palliative care was called for. Who did it, whether or not it was well done, and whatever its effects should now be past history. It is only when all was badly handled that it should colour the quality and effectiveness of communication in palliative care.

Communications between the doctor and relatives

It cannot be stated strongly enough that the needs of the relatives (and other carers) are not the same as the needs of the patient, self-evident as that may be. The relatives usually feel sad, angry, frightened, helpless and unskilled, apprehensive, increasingly tired and very lonely. At any other time in life they would probably be able to speak of these feelings to their loved one or another member of the family, but if that is the patient, or everyone else in the family is feeling the same, they have no one to whom they can turn. The isolation and helplessness is something they have probably never experienced before. To make matters worse, the burden of caring often lands on relatives who may themselves be elderly and unwell.

All this is very stressful, but even that is not the whole picture. The strain is made worse by the 'conspiracy of silence', the great effort made to keep the awful truth from the patient (who, experience shows, probably knows all there is to know about his condition but has not disclosed any of that insight to his family). Few of us are good actors and actresses, so maintaining this charade soon exhausts the carer.

Finally, a feature of our age, the family is usually scattered. Members reappear after being lost or distant for years, possibly feeling guilty but eager to make amends by throwing their weight around 'organizing'. Within a day of arriving, they demand to see the doctor and discuss every aspect of the care, or go to the hospital to ensure that everything has been done which should have been done, often stirring up unpleasant feelings in siblings and rarely contributing much to the care. Harmony within the family would be so helpful, but at times like that feels elusive.

Some key points with regard to communicating with relatives:

◆ The patient must always be the focus of our care, no matter how demanding the relatives and great their problems. The family doctor is, however, in a unique position to help the relatives, because some may be his patients, people he has known for years. Ultimately, however, everything must be said primarily for the good of the patient.

◆ Relatives need regularly updated information about the patient rather than simply the diagnosis and proposed treatment which is usually given to them at the beginning. A common complaint is that they were not keep up to date, even though the patient was well informed. It is easy to brief them on the patient's care without helping them to fully understand either the rationale behind the treatment or the advanced nature of the illness.

◆ Relatives need different information from that which the patient needs.

  • There is the information needed to enable them to care for the patient; for example, about diet, exercise, medication, things to be on the lookout for, and so on.

  • They also need information and help to enable them to cope with this sad and frightening experience. Put another way, they need to be cared for and have their needs recognized and respected. Many say they appreciated how well the doctors looked after the patient but feel that they, the relatives and carers, were inadvertently neglected.

Some examples may make this clearer. They need to be asked about their sleep, how tired they are, how well they feel they are coping, and whether any additional help would be appreciated. They need to be able to articulate their fears and apprehensions, foolish as they may sound to others, fears surrounding bleeding, choking, fits, sudden death, and how they will recognize death when it happens.

♦ It has to be remembered that relatives may have emotions they are too embarrassed or upset to mention. Being able to talk about them to the family doctor or nurse can be most helpful. For example, they may have lost all love for each other years before the terminal illness and now find it difficult to keep up a pretence of affection and sadness. ('I'm not a good enough actress to pretend I love him when I don't.') Another has been happily married but now feels that his wife with marked personality change as a result of the glioma is not really his wife. ('I feel I'm looking after a complete stranger, doctor.') There is the lady who cares for her husband in coma for months and wants the doctor to understand why she cannot cry as people seem to expect her to. ('I've no tears left. In a sense I lost him months ago but people don't seem to understand that.') There is the person totally lacking in confidence, who has never needed to cope on her own, whose every thought is about how she will survive without her husband. ('Thank goodness you understand how apprehensive I am, doctor. Everyone else thinks I'm heartless.') To use the modern jargon, relatives need permission to be themselves!

♦ Even family doctors can overlook the societal pressures on relatives. Relatives may be determined to keep the patient at home as long as possible but everyone they speak to expresses surprise and asks why they have not insisted on hospital or hospice admission. They meet those who try to tell them that if the patient had been under a different doctor things would have been better, or hint that the patient would at least get parenteral nutrition or fluids if the family doctor arranged admission. Some of the opiophobia we encounter is flamed by the neighbour or visitor who expresses shock that the doctor has started the patient on morphine because, as they point out, it seems such a shame to make a man an addict in his final weeks of life! It is often worth exploring what people are saying to them or what family members are suggesting.

♦ Apprehension about the future is normal for relatives but talk about it not always socially acceptable. However, when the doctor or nurse mention it, it becomes respectable and acceptable, especially when they may be the only people, including the family, who ever do. We make a grave mistake as professional carers if we think that all their grief relates to the present. Some of it relates to the past and their regrets, but much to the unknown future looming ahead. Will there be money problems, how will they cope with bills, who will show them how to write cheques, and, in the near future, how will they organize a funeral? Reasonable anxieties, but dare they admit to them and who will listen and help?

We suggest that a similar 'technique' be employed whether speaking to patients or relatives. Clearly signify that you will try to help two separate though related people, the patient and the relative(s). 'First tell me about you—every little detail please no matter how trivial anything might sound! I want to know exactly how you're feeling. After we've talked about you and I've tried to answer all your questions we'll talk about your wife, shall we?' That is said to the patient. A similar thing is said to the relative, whether in the house or at the surgery. 'I'll talk to John first (the patient) and do what I can for him, then, if I may I'll have a chat with you (the relative) and hear how you are and if there is anything you want to know or I can do for you.'

Finally, and perhaps surprisingly, the time comes when the questions get fewer, and less and less is said provided the doctor and nurse have reiterated time after time that they are ready to answer questions or explain anything. Eventually the time comes, particularly when the care is being given in the home, that they just leave everything in the hands of the doctor and nurse whom they have come to trust completely. 'I trust you all completely—if there's something I ought to know I know you'll tell me.' 'Success' is when the patient says he or she feels 'safe'!

Communicating with fellow professionals

Stop and ask the question—'what does he/she need to know about this patient?' This applies whether we are writing to a consultant or preparing for a team meeting with nurses and partners. It applies whether the question is being asked by a nurse or a doctor, by a social worker or a pastoral care worker. Our aim should be to give as much information as is necessary (but no more) to enable the colleague to contribute as well as they possibly can. Gratuitous information is useless and time wasting. The problem is that few of us know exactly the skills and potential contribution of our colleagues and many of us enjoy displaying our own skills.

Hospital colleagues

If you do not know how much information colleagues need, then ask them! If you want a colleague to send you all the relevant information you need, politely tell him so that he will know for the future. The only caveat is that many hospitals use 'model' letters to guide junior doctors and the family doctor may have to put up with that, but gently remind the consultant that one of the things he most values is information on what the patient was told and how he reacted. That very crucial information is probably not in the model, although all the biochemistry is certain to be listed.

The ideal, of course, is not to depend on letters but to have more conversations with hospital colleagues, even if they have to be over the telephone. There seems no easy way to achieve this ideal. Family doctors, for their part, might be prepared to dedicate a time when they could be contacted, say at the end of the morning or afternoon surgery.

Key information which should be sought from hospitals includes:

- the consultant's overall view of the present condition of the patient and recommendations about treatment and care
- the results (and possibly their significance) of recent investigations
- details of what the patient has been told and what the patient said, asked, and was told
- details of anything which might happen that the family doctor should be alert for
- follow-up arrangements

Team colleagues

Members of the primary care health team need information for two different scenarios; the day-to-day care and the occasional house-call when it is likely to be a different doctor and/or nurse who attends and need as much information as possible.

Arrangements have to be in place for regular, possibly informal meetings between the regular doctor and nurse. They need only last minutes, recounting details of the last visit, changes in condition or medication, things to be on the lookout for, and 'who does what'.

Both doctors and nurses sometimes forget how much detail a nurse needs when caring for the palliative care patient—the doctor perhaps does not think to pass on that information and the nurse perhaps lacks the confidence to ask for it. For example, it is insufficient for a doctor merely to report that a patient has a bronchogenic carcinoma. If he tells his colleague it is a squamous carcinoma, then she will then be alerted to the possibility of hypercalcaemia and be on the lookout for features of it.

If he tells the nurse that the patient has a small cell carcinoma, then she will know that some of them eventually metastasize to the brain and will be alerted to features of raised intracranial pressure.

At the weekly team meeting the regular doctor and nurse must update all the colleagues, particularly about problems looming up, possible problems or even emergencies they may have to handle, and their plans for the care of the patient (staying at home, extra help planned, admission to such-and-such unit, etc.)

Possibly more important than anything else is that when an explanation has been given by any member of the team to the patient or family, the colleagues in the primary care team should be told the details. The reason is perhaps obvious. One person's illustration intended to explain something is another's conundrum. Soon people are speaking of how two doctors (or two nurses) never say the same thing.

Nurse-to-nurse communications

Sad to say, communications between nurses are sometimes as bad as between doctors or between doctors and nurses.

Patients and relatives often pay more attention to what nurses say and advise than they do to what doctors say, which often they cannot understand. It is therefore essential that visiting nurses are seen to be saying the same thing. Perhaps there is no such thing as a casual remark in palliative care, but much damage is done by them. 'He's probably being sick because of his morphine' is such a remark. If the patient is still in the first few days of opioid medication, the comment may be right. If not, and if there was ever any hesitation about taking the morphine, the seeds of doubt and anxiety have been sown.

Confusion is frequently created by different nurses using different treatment regimens and not conferring with each other. Once again, some illustrations may help here. Without finding out what laxative routine a patient is on, and knowing why it has been chosen, a deputizing nurse can visit a patient and give an unnecessary enema or suppository. An even more common event is for one nurse to apply her favourite dressing only to have the next nurse apply a different dressing the following day. No information is too small or 'trivial' to pass on.

In all communications, whether between doctors, doctors and nurses, or between nurses, it is so reassuring to patients and relatives to hear that details are being passed on between them. This cannot be overstated. It is something they tell you has helped them to develop trust in their attendants. 'Yes, doctor was telling me how much that new pill has helped but

I said I would pop in and see how your bowels are. Wasn't that good news about your last X-ray results? Dr Black said you were pleased.'

Does it need to be said? In all communications, and particularly written ones, remember to add a word of thanks. Try to end even the most business-like, clinical letter to a hospital colleague with something along the lines of '. . . and many thanks for all your help looking after this gentleman' or ' . . . thanks for such a helpful letter.' When it is the team doing the caring, allude to that in the letter '. . . my nursing colleagues and I appreciate being able to discuss this lady with you like this.'

9

Home, hospital, or hospice?

In this chapter we shall look at the pros and cons of being cared for, and dying, in one's home, in a hospital, or in a hospice. The subject is much more complicated than would at first appear. Nevertheless, it is a question which usually cannot be avoided.

What can we learn from research on the subject? Staying at home as long as possible and dying at home are not the same thing. It seems that most patients want to be at home as long as that is feasible (something we shall return to) but fewer than expected actually want to die in their own beds. Research also shows that, much as relatives will say they want to care for the patient at home, they do not want a death in the home and are actually hoping for admission before the patient asks for it. Finally, research seems to suggest that whether or not a patient dies in his own bed does not depend on the number of professionals coming into the home, but on the quality of care being offered there, both to the patient and to the carers. That, after all, is one reason why this book has been produced.

Home

Here we are thinking of the patient's home, or the home of a friend or relative. We are not referring to a 'nursing home'.

What are the positive points in favour of care at home?

- Home is usually a place of memories, happiness, love, safety, and familiarity.

- Home is where relatives also feel familiar with everything, where they can feel relaxed and confident.

- Home is where care is provided by the family doctor and his/her nursing colleagues, perhaps all known to the patient and family for years and years. Again, familiarity and safety.

What are the negative features about care at home?

◆ The house or apartment may be small. Many people may live in it, affording little privacy for the patient and little space for the additional furniture and equipment that may have to be brought in. Family members may be very inconvenienced and even frightened when a person is critically ill there.

◆ Facilities may be frankly inadequate for sick nursing. There may be no hot water. Toilet facilities may have to be shared with many others. Smells from the kitchen may permeate through to the room where the patient is and, on occasions, unpleasant odours from the patient may reach other rooms. There may be noise and no peace to sleep.

◆ The family members, whether they can articulate this or not, may be frightened by having a seriously ill person in the house, very near to them or even in the same room, knowing that he will die. In our modern Western society very few people have seen death before their fifties and the many deaths they have witnessed on television or in films have usually been traumatic and profoundly disturbing, quite different from what we have learnt to expect as a result of modern palliative care.

In short, home is familiar and full of rich memories, safe when there are no crises but not ideal when things go wrong or the rest of the family look as though they are not coping well.

Hospital

What type of a hospital are we speaking about? A large university teaching hospital, a district general hospital, or a little community hospital staffed by local family doctors and nurses who live nearby, all well recognized and respected in the local community?

University teaching hospital

We are all familiar with them. They may be vast and impersonal, noisy and frightening, but it is probably in one of them that our patient received the specialist treatment which has kept him or her going longer than was ever thought possible, with chemotherapy, or dialysis, or whatever. Some of the nursing staff never seem to change and always remember you when you go back, although it is true that you seldom see the same doctor twice and in some hospitals you seem never to see the consultant.

You can be sure the equipment is there and is as good as money can buy. If there was a crisis, there would be specialists able to help you and the equipment they needed to do so. Very reassuring, especially when you have had one or two emergencies in the past year.

Although many of the specialist units are to be found in hospital, there may not be a bed available if you are admitted urgently. The result is that you may land up in a totally unfamiliar ward with no faces you recognize and doctors and nurses who may know nothing about your disease or about palliative care. Having said that, increasing numbers of large hospitals now have Hospital Palliative Care teams operating in them, seeing patients in every corner of the hospital. They take referrals from all specialties and it is very helpful if the family doctor especially asks in the referring letter for them to be called in to his patient on admission.

In short, abundant medical, nursing, and diagnostic expertise and equipment are available—very reassuring in crises, but sometimes seen as less caring and intimate when the priority is for the highest quality palliative care in the final weeks of life.

District general hospital

For the sake of readers not familiar with the British hospital model it should be explained that a district general hospital (DGH) is a hospital of 300–500 beds, staffed by surgeons and physicians of high calibre but not claiming to specialist expertise within their disciplines, and usually without specialist units. A DGH may teach undergraduate and postgraduate students but is not an officially affiliated department of a university. It must not be thought that a DGH is a second-class hospital. The standard of care is of the highest but it does not claim to be a tertiary referral unit. Its physicians will each have specialties in which they have a particular interest but they will see patients with any condition. Likewise the nursing care is excellent but there are not usually clinical nurse specialists or nurse practitioners. There may, however, be a Hospital Palliative Care team and, if the referring general practitioner knows this, he should request that his patient be seen by the team as soon as possible after admission.

Because a DGH serves a small area, the local community becomes familiar with it and often has a sense of ownership. It feels less daunting that a city-based university teaching hospital with all its tertiary hospital expertise and academics.

Nursing homes

Nursing homes mean different things in different countries. In the United Kingdom they are usually small, run by nurses though often part of a commercial chain, and primarily for long-stay patients, usually more frail than ill, needing more attention than they can receive in their own homes. Few of the nurses have had training in modern palliative care, although this is being corrected in many local and national training programmes. Medical care is, without exception in the United Kingdom, provided by the patient's own family doctor.

In some countries nursing homes resemble private hospitals more than cosy homes. They are real alternatives to small hospitals and sometimes employ their own doctors.

For the palliative care patient the benefits of a nursing home are that it is small, homely, and probably not difficult to access for visiting relatives. It is ideal when the needs are primarily nursing, with few, if any, complex medical problems.

The disadvantages of nursing homes are the lack of nursing expertise in palliative care (and often no knowledge whatsoever of pain management, the opioids, and many of the drugs used in this care) and the often poorly defined relationship with the doctor. There is also, of course, the expense, most nursing homes being costly.

Hospice or palliative care unit

It is crucially important that the doctor caring for a palliative care patient knows as much as possible about his or her local hospice or palliative care unit. They vary greatly.

The smaller hospices, usually with 5–10 beds, are staffed by nurses, many of whom will have had palliative care training. The medical input will usually be from a local practice, often a doctor who has made a special study of palliative care. Most hospices will have part-time physiotherapists and occupational therapists, and benefit from visits from local clergy. Smaller hospices usually take patients with malignant disease and a few will accept those with motor neurone disease.

The larger hospices, though still using that name, will probably be specialist palliative care units characterized by their senior doctors being consultants in palliative medicine (or specialist registrars in training), and there being junior doctors as well. All senior nurses will have undertaken advanced training, and even have degrees, in palliative care nursing. There will also be a complement of professions allied to medicine (PAMs) equally experienced in this work. In addition to the in-patient facility there will usually be a Home Care Service offering advice and support for patients at home, a Day Unit, a Hospital Palliative Care Team, an education department, and a research unit. Most will accept patients with any pathology, although the bulk of patients will have malignant disease. It is worth knowing that the average length of stay in a specialist palliative care unit is 2 weeks or less, with up to 60 per cent of patients being discharged home.

None of these details should be read as criticisms of hospices and palliative care units. They all have their place in the spectrum of care provision. Clearly, however, they are different and it is these differences that affect the doctor's decision when referring a patient to them.

♦ When the needs are primarily nursing and there are few problems for which medical expertise is needed, or thought likely to be needed, then the patient will benefit from a hospice.

♦ When there are difficult-to-control symptoms and/or major psychosocial problems, then the combined expertise and experience of the specialist palliative care unit's staff are called for, provided that it is remembered that few, if any, such units accept long-stay patients.

Keeping a patient at home

Research and experience seem to show that patients are happy to be cared for at home provided four conditions are met.

♦ The quality of pain and symptom control is excellent.

♦ The patient can see that the relatives are also being cared for.

♦ Emergencies are handled with skill.

♦ Admission to hospital, hospice, or palliative care unit can be arranged at short notice if home care breaks down for any reason.

They may appear self-evident but are important. The public is becoming increasingly aware of how good care can be and, rightly, will not tolerate poorly controlled pain or any other distress. They increasingly expect that the patient will be seen at home by a palliative care specialist, whether doctor or nurse, or be admitted somewhere.

The vast experience accumulated by hospice home-care services has demonstrated that patients are very aware of the suffering of their relatives. Many agree to admission for that reason alone, although they never admit to that in front of the loved ones. Emergencies may not be regarded as such by the family doctor or nurse but are seen as such by the patient. They include such events as an escalation of pain, urinary retention, an acute paranoid or confusional state, or something as 'trivial' as hiccups that prevents sleep. Any failure to provide immediate skilled handling of each crisis soon leads to admission. Having a 'safety net' in the form of ready admission to the hospice within a day or two of asking for a place is undoubtedly reassuring to all concerned.

In this chapter it is assumed that the doctor and nurse are skilled and experienced in home care, although not necessarily in palliative care. They already know how to enlist additional help in the form of domestic help (Home Helps in the UK, Home Makers in North America), night nurses, physiotherapists who will visit homes, modifications to the house and sick room arranged by the occupational therapists, and even special laundry services in many parts of the country.

To provide high-quality palliative care in the home they may wish to make use of:

♦ the local hospice/palliative care home-care service, for additional advice and support;

♦ specialist nurses such as Macmillan and Marie Curie;

♦ special equipment available on loan from the hospice/palliative care unit or, in the UK, the Red Cross;

♦ home visits by the local palliative medicine consultant, failing which, phone advice can be helpful.

Reasons for considering admission

It must be stressed that admission need not be for terminal care with no possibility of discharge home again. Most units, whether hospital, hospice, or palliative care, will gladly admit for a few days to bring a symptom under control, rationalize medication, or give the relatives a break. There is much to be said for such short-term admissions. They reassure patients that something can always be done to help, that people do in fact come out of hospices, and they make the final admission that bit easier because the hospital or hospice is familiar. Here we shall look first at short-term admissions:

♦ difficult-to-control suffering, whether physical or psychosocial;

♦ recurring 'crises' in the home;

- as a respite for relatives, although usually they deny the need for such respite.

Where should the patient be admitted?

The simple answer is where the patient will get the most appropriate care and feel most at home and safe. It largely depends on what the doctor and nurse feel are the key problems affecting the patient at home. Some examples will illustrate this.

- If skilled nursing care is needed, as for example to heal a pressure sore, deal with an offensive fungating tumour, or restore appetite, then the most appropriate place will be the local hospice. If there is an unusual pain, or intractable vomiting, or features suggestive of hypercalcaemia, then skilled medical input is needed. Admission should therefore be to the nearest specialist palliative care unit. If ascites has developed, or a pleural effusion is embarrassing breathing, the doctor must know whether the palliative care unit is happy to drain them (or even perform pleurodesis) or whether it is better to have the patient readmitted to the oncology or chest ward. Much will depend on the doctor's prior knowledge of what each service can offer. As at any other time in general practice, the doctor will try to match his patient with the colleague and unit best suited to the patient.

- There are some patients who might benefit from admission to the hospice but feel they are 'not at that stage'. On the other hand, they are very content to be readmitted to the oncology ward where they have been before or to a general medical ward. If that happens, the doctor must be totally explicit with his hospital colleagues about the reasons for admission and what he hopes will be done for the patient. If this is not done, the patient may be subjected to further batteries of tests and investigations, inappropriate at this time.

Reasons for admission for terminal care

There is usually a confluence of reasons leading to the patient being transferred from home to somewhere else to die. Very seldom is it 'simply' poor symptom control. In fact, relatives often request admission just when the patient has been made more comfortable than he or she has been for a long time.

Sometimes the terminal phase is longer than relatives had been led to expect or programmed themselves for. Often friends and neighbours bring subliminal pressure to bear on them. Sometimes it is the patient who suggests it, perhaps because he dreads dying at home, or wants to shield loved ones, or sees what a strain it is proving to be.

In a sense the 'reason' is not as important as the preparation needed by the patient and the family. The patient needs to be reassured about the quality of care they will get. The relatives need to feel they have made the right decision, one they will never live to regret, and that they have done well at home. This is critically important. Years later, family members will recount how impressed the doctor was with how they coped at home. It is essential that the doctor and nurse, and the family they are trying to support, are honest with the patient. They must not hide behind euphemisms such as 'see if they can help your pain and get you home as quickly as possible' or ' just a few days and we'll have you home' when they and the patient know this is not true. At times like that the patient deserves honesty. There is much to be said for one of the hospice or specialist palliative care staff coming to the home to see the patient and establish trust before the patient is admitted.

Where should the patient be admitted for terminal care?

Sad to say, the doctor may not have much choice. A busy oncology ward, or indeed a busy general hospital, may not be willing to accept somebody for terminal care. Many do not see that as their responsibility even though they have known the patient for some time.

- If there is the slightest chance of difficult care problems arising, the referral must be to the specialist palliative care unit so that they can be dealt with on the spot and not necessitate transfer elsewhere.
- Otherwise arrange admission as near the patient's home and relatives as possible, making visiting easier.

While fully recognizing that it may often be impossible, it has to be said that there are few things more comforting and cheering for a terminally ill person than being visited by their own doctor or nurse, whether at home, in the hospital, or in the local hospice/palliative care unit. As a patient once said to one of the authors 'There are times when you need doctors with all those letters after their name. There are times when you need a friend because you are so lonely. It is wonderful at this time in life when your doctor has become your friend.'

Some final thoughts about where patients can be looked after and where they may die.

Patients tell us that they feel a total loss of control over their lives as they get frailer. It upsets them greatly. They are not always told why they are being treated here or admitted there. They are expected to leave such decisions to doctor. Perhaps this reflects medical paternalism or perhaps just our reluctance to ask the patient to make difficult decisions when they are so ill. However, it seems to be important that they know that we hope to keep them at home, know why we may have to revise that plan, and that we are looking far into the future and planning accordingly. Dying is frightening enough without having to worry about who will look after you and where that will be.

Never make firm, inflexible plans but be prepared to change them as the patient's needs and wishes change, as they always do. The person who insists on remaining at home may soon be so frightened there that he asks for admission, and vice versa. The relative who says that nothing will come in the way of keeping the loved one at home may be the first to ask for admission, often long before the doctor had thought much about it.

In palliative care the relatives almost always claim to know exactly what the patient is experiencing and wanting. The wise doctor and nurse always listen to the close relatives but then balance what they have heard with what they have been told by the patient and have seen with their own eyes. Research has shown that relatives always see the patient as having more pain and anxiety than is the case. However, their assessment of other suffering is usually accurate and reliable.

Wherever the patient is cared for, and wherever he or she dies, always reassure the relatives that what was done was for the patient's good and their decisions have been the right ones. They have probably not done any of this before and need to be reassured that they performed well. There is little doubt that their subsequent grief is modestly reduced when they know that their caring was commended by the professionals.

10

Nursing Issues at Home

Despite an increasing trend for death to occur in institutions, terminally ill patients spend most of their time at home. Enabling patients to have a choice about the place of care demands an integrated approach to care by the many different health care professionals. This chapter outlines the issues that need to be addressed to achieve high-quality palliative care at home.

Assessment of the home

The home environment may need modification to allow the patient to be cared for at home. The community nurse, occupational therapist, and physiotherapist usually carry out the assessment. A social worker may also give valuable input to home assessments in supporting families, arranging packages of care, and with financial advice. Primary care teams are best placed to help patients and families to express their wishes and to be involved in planning care.

Aids, appliances, and equipment

Practical home modifications

Baby listeners	Liquidizer
Bath aids	Radio/TV tapes
Commode	Rails
Communication aids	Ramps
Creating bedroom downstairs	Showers
Cushions/pressure-relieving mattresses	Stair lift
Fans	Table
Hoist	Toilet appliances

Hospital bed	Wheelchair
Incontinence supplies	Widened doors
Laptop trays	

Co-ordination of home care

General practitioners and district nurses are the key professionals responsible for medical and nursing care at home and should be the first professionals consulted when planning a discharge from hospital. If the hospital team feel that specialist palliative care is indicated, they should discuss this with the primary care team before involving clinical nurse specialists or community specialist teams. It is important that members of the primary care team are aware of the skills of the specialist community palliative care teams.

Clinical nurse specialists

Macmillan nurses

These nurses have expertise in advising on pain and symptom control, monitoring drug changes and side-effects, and explaining treatments to patients and families. They have a much smaller caseload than community nurses and so they can give time to patients and, equally importantly, their carers. Clinical nurse specialists are also a source of professional support to community nurses and general practitioners. Clinical nurse specialists can advise on financial allowances and grants available to patients and families. In summary, these nurses complement the services provided by the primary care team.

Marie Curie nurses

Marie Curie nurses may be of a range of nursing grades and are available to give hands-on care. They usually, but not exclusively, are available at night to give carers some respite. The availability of this service varies enormously from area to area in the UK and doctors must familiarize themselves with their local situation.

Communication between professionals

If the patient is being discharged from hospital, it is vital that the primary care teams have detailed information about the diagnosis, prognosis, aims of care, drug treatments, and details of what has been said to the patient and family.

Completing the community nursing record, which remains in the patient's home, can facilitate communication between professionals in the home.

Packages of care

Social workers are generally responsible for co-ordinating the package of care at home, which involves the primary care team home-care assistance, specialist palliative care, and non-professional voluntary support. These various agencies need to be carefully co-ordinated to provide care to meet the assessed needs of the patient and family.

Anticipating needs

The problem for some family doctors looking after patients with advanced disease is to know who to refer and for what indications. If there is any doubt in referring a patient, it is useful to discuss the problems with a palliative medicine specialist.

Out-patient clinics

These may be useful when a specialist assessment of a particular problem is required. Patients receiving palliative care want to be looked after by their general practitioner at home. There is therefore a need for rapid access for specialist advice. Patients do not need to attend hospital clinics just to monitor progression of their disease.

Hospice day care

This can provide a day out for the patient and respite for the carer. Provision of Day Hospice care varies; some have a medical bias and others are nurse-led and yet others focus on diversion, relaxation, and complementary therapies.

One almost has to see a Day Hospice in order to appreciate its uniquely positive atmosphere, otherwise it could sound negative and morbid if one remembers that all attending have advanced life-threatening illnesses. The atmosphere is always relaxed and informal and as homely as it possibly can be. Contrary to what might be thought, its aim is not to divert the patient's attention from the seriousness of their condition but rather to focus on what can be done to improve the quality of their life. Activities are skilfully tailored to each person's needs and abilities. Some just want to sit and watch, others to talk or be entertained, whilst most relish developing old hobbies or skills or even taking on something quite new.

The casual visitor will find it difficult to realize just how ill these people are, for all around is activity, laughter, and living.

It has rightly been said that Day Hospices are not a preparation for dying but a reaffirmation of living. The benefits extend far beyond the patient. Caring relatives are released from their duties for a few hours to do shopping, visit the hairdresser, or just to do nothing. The 'death and dying stigma' of the hospice is erased and soon patient and relatives come to regard it as a positive place rather than one to be feared.

Primary care team members need to learn how to best use local Day Hospice facilities. They can identify those who need the offer to be taken out of their homes to have a break and to meet others. Often patients who are isolated and have become introspective and morbid benefit most from the positive support available at the Day Hospice. Relatives too need a well-earned break if they are to be enabled to continue to care.

Pain clinic

The pain clinic is an out-patient facility usually under the direction of specially trained anaesthetists, supported where possible by clinical psychologists, radiologists, and physiotherapists. In addition to working with sophisticated nerve-blocking procedures, much of their work is skilled diagnosis of intractable pain problems. Adjuvant analgesics and psychological techniques are used to assist the patients.

Community physiotherapy

Incredibly, there are still some who feel that physiotherapy has little to offer the terminally ill patient. One reason is possibly that they have not considered the benefits until the patient is too frail to make use of them! As so often in palliative care, the earlier the referral the better.

The physiotherapist has a particularly important role in managing breathlessness in palliative care. They can teach patients how to relax, to improve their breathing, and to expectorate. Patients and relatives can be shown better ways of transferring from bed/chair to commode or toilet, how to walk with appropriate aids, and how to have an improved quality of life by being able to maximize their abilities.

Apart from this vital role in helping patients with reduced mobility from breathlessness, weakness, and fatigue, or from cord compression, physiotherapists can help with the management of lymphoedema.

Complementary therapies

There is a bewildering choice of complementary therapies available. The following suggestions reflect the authors' views. Complementary therapies which achieve and help relaxation and which do not have any harmful side-effects are generally acceptable. Amongst those that are becoming more established are the following.

Acupuncture

Acupuncture has a real place in palliative care. A palliative medicine consultant or a pain specialist may recommend it and its benefits are proven for a few conditions such as in the control of pain and nausea.

Hypnotherapy

Hypnotherapy also has a role in palliative care. Performed by a medical hypnotherapist with appropriate qualifications, hypnosis is a useful technique to teach patients to enable them to relax. Its use as a psychotherapeutic tool is more controversial in palliative care.

Aromatherapy

Aromatherapy is increasingly learned and practised by many in palliative care who are convinced of its benefits. It is certainly a useful relaxation technique.

If complementary therapies are available and administered by experienced practitioners with appropriate qualifications, then these should be offered to patients who are then free to make up their own mind. The emphasis should be that these therapies are complementary to conventional medicine and should not be viewed as an alternative. If a patient wants to try an unproven complementary therapy, provided it will not harm the patient, they should be allowed to do so, and reminded that this will not harm the doctor–patient relationship—the GP is still there for them.

Informal carers—family and friends

Patients need the support of family and friends if they are to remain at home. These informal carers also have a variety of needs. Carers needs include information about the patient, the patient's illness, what resources are available to help, education about how to care for the patient, and psychosocial support for themselves.

Carers, like everyone else, find uncertainty difficult to bear. If patient's carers are informed, then they can be involved in decision making. Doctors must avoid setting up situations of collusion by informing carers and not the patient.

Some carers want to be involved in simple nursing and they should receive help and education from community nurses to do this. Simple mouth care, feeding, and administration of drugs are all areas where carers can be involved. Professionals also need to respect those carers who are not able to carry out nursing tasks—we should not make assumptions about their abilities.

Carers require psychosocial support. Anxiety and depression are common among informal carers. Professionals can find out about carers' problems by asking questions about the impact of the patient's illness on their life and how they are feeling. Carers should be encouraged to express their concerns and fears and doctors must be prepared to see beyond the brave face. Carers are often reluctant to discuss their needs because they do not wish to be judged inadequate and they do not want to put themselves before the needs of the patient. However, many dying patients admitted to hospital could be cared for at home if informal carers were given better support.

Home nursing issues

Mouth care

Mouth problems can stop the patient from drinking and eating. Assessment of oral hygiene is an essential part of care. The important issues to address are detailed in Chapter 2.

Skin care

Patients at risk of pressure sores need careful monitoring and daily inspection of pressure areas. Special pressure-relieving mattresses are sometimes needed. If pain is present, gel or colloid dressings can be left in place for several days. The topical application of benzydamine to the edges of an ulcer can be of help. If changing a dressing is painful then rapid-acting morphine may be given 20 minutes before the dressing is changed.

Malodour may be relieved either with topical metronidazole gel or systemic metronidazole 400 milligrams twice a day.

Nutrition is important from an early stage, because good hydration and a mixed diet will encourage healing. However, at a later stage, patients should eat what they like rather than adhering to a strict dietary regimen.

Faecal and urinary contamination require specific treatments because if pressure sores are contaminated in this way they will not heal.

The psychological aspects of treating pressure sores/malignant ulcers always need to be addressed. Patients are likely to become withdrawn and depressed and should be given a chance to discuss their fears in a sensitive and compassionate way.

Lymphoedema

Lymphoedema is a result of reduced lymphatic drainage, either caused by lymphatic obstruction due to tumour infection or as a consequence of surgical or radiotherapy treatments. Patients may complain of stiffness, a heavy or bursting feeling, or pain from related conditions such as cellulitis. It is important to attend to skin care to prevent infection and treat infections such as cellulitis quickly with suitable antibiotics.

Lymphoedema may affect any limb but is much commoner in the arms, due to the large numbers of patients with breast cancer who have axillary surgery or radiotherapy. Although usually unilateral, it can be bilateral. In almost all cases it is a complication of breast carcinoma and its treatment by radiotherapy and/or radical surgery, although the latter is now rare. It is important to remember that it is not a terminal event, often developing months or even years before the terminal phase is entered. It is difficult to overstate how distressing it can be for sufferers. Not only is the arm unsightly but it is difficult to get clothes to fit it, there is often neuropathic pain, and it can be so heavy that the patient develops spinal problems trying to correct postural problems caused by it. Patients sometimes say they feel they are attached to the affected arm rather than vice versa. Appropriate management from its earliest days is imperative if the patient is to be spared much misery.

Management

There is no doubt that the best course of action is to refer the patient to the nearest lymphoedema clinic. If one is not known in the locality then contact the nearest specialist palliative care unit where they may offer the expert services of a physiotherapist trained in lymphoedema care or will advise where to get expert help.

Until a few years ago the therapy consisted of arm pumps, at first simple and then made more sophisticated and sequential, but in recent years remarkable results have been obtained by a short-stretch multilayer bandage accompanied by special lymphoedema massage on the contralateral side. Lymphorrhoea requires referral to a specialist palliative care team for assessment, antibiotic treatment, and specialized bandaging.

There is no place for diuretics in treating lymphoedema, although they may be used to relieve any accompanying pitting oedema.

One final word of warning. Do not attribute bilateral arm oedema to lymphoedema until you have excluded superior vena caval obstruction.

Nutrition

Feeding an ill person is a basic human urge and time needs to be spent explaining to patients and relatives that a patient with advanced cancer and cachexia–anorexia syndrome is not dying of starvation.

It is sometimes helpful to be able to demonstrate to relatives that the patient is not hungry and anorexia is a consequence of the disease rather than a cause of the cachexia. However, if the patient is unable to swallow, for example due to an oesophageal tumour, and is complaining of hunger, enteral feeding may need consideration, and a gastrostomy feeding tube may be of benefit.

In managing this anorexia–cachexia, the doctor and nurse need to address the significance of diet to the patient and relatives and what advice to give.

The concerns of patients and relatives

There are many myths surrounding diet and nutrition and these need to be dispelled:

◆ Without food we die, or, if we eat we live.

When a patient has reached the stage of far-advanced malignancy with cachexia, the body can no longer metabolize food to increase lean body mass or fat. Intensive nutrition only has a small place in rare situations when patients are recovering from surgery and awaiting further aggressive active treatments such as chemotherapy and is futile in the patient with terminal cancer cachexia.

It requires considerable skill and patience to explain to relatives that the patient will no longer benefit from these measures. They need to understand that a reduced food intake or the withdrawal of parenteral nutrition is not meant to shorten life but is a recognition that life is coming to an end because of the underlying disease, not because of medically sanctioned starvation.

◆ Some foods can heal cancer

The food that a patient takes in the terminal stage should be what the patient is able to enjoy. Small portions of foods that they fancy are of much more benefit than vitamin supplements, proprietary high-calorie nutritional supplements, or bizarre diets including agents like hydrazine or carrot juice.

◆ Diets need to be complicated

At the terminal stage of the illness the simple advice to 'give him what he fancies when he wants it' can frighten relatives by its simplicity. This simple truth seems too good to be true.

Patients need clear advice from the doctors and nurses to reassure them that there are not certain foods which have specific healing or therapeutic qualities and nor is there any need to undergo complicated dietary regimes. The following dietary guidelines are offered.

Dietary guidelines

When a patient is in the final weeks of life the following may be noted:

◆ The patient will vary from day to day in what he wants, how much he will take, and when he takes it. Some days he may eat well, but the following day may eat nothing. This is quite normal but needs to be explained.

◆ He may eat more in the morning and almost nothing in the evening.

◆ The nearer the patient is to death the more he will prefer fluids. These may be icy cold or in some cases very hot.

◆ The patient will know what is best. Small portions of fairly bland foods, avoiding spices, are often appreciated. Patients do not need high roughage diets.

When the explanation is given to the patient and carers together, it relieves the tension which often exists when carers are forcing food onto a patient, only to have it rejected.

In summary, dietary advice for these patients and their caring families is simple and straightforward. The feelings and fears of both patients and relatives need to be discussed.

Fungating tumours and odours

The discharge and smell from a fungating lesion can be embarrassing for the patient and test the love and determination of the most caring relative. It has to be remembered, however, that the tumour may be relatively slow growing. If the patient is admitted to hospital or palliative care unit it should not be for long but rather for respite for the family and an opportunity to try new dressings and topical preparations on the patient. There are so many proprietary dressings available that no attempt will be made here to discuss or evaluate them.

Capillary bleeding can be reduced by applying

- proprietary haemostatic dressings
- silver nitrate soaks applied daily in a strength of 1:5000, made up specially and kept in a dark bottle
- adrenalin soaks in a strength of 1:1000
- alum paste 1 per cent applied directly on the bleeding site
- Oxycel or Polycel gauze applied to the site (not widely prescribable but sometimes obtainable from a hospital operating theatre)
- bismuth subnitrate/iodoform paste (BIPP) applied generously on gauze and left undisturbed for 3–4 days.

Malodour can be reduced with

- metronidazole gel applied directly to the site
- metronidazole tablets
- bismuth subnitrate/iodoform paste as described above
- activated charcoal pads applied on top of, not under, all other dressings on the affected site are usually highly effective
- frequent dressing changes, often more than once a day

Exudation can be reduced with

- proprietary absorbent dressings

It is important to remember that radiotherapy has an important role here. The advice of a radiation oncologist should be sought about fungating tumours, bleeding sites, and exudation.

Dying at home

If the death is anticipated, the patient and family have an opportunity to discuss this. Recent guidelines have been produced which summarize the important issues that may face the patient, and which need to be addressed to achieve death with dignity.

- To know when death is coming and to understand what can be expected
- To be able to retain control of what happens
- To be afforded dignity and privacy
- To have control over pain relief and other symptom control
- To have choice and control over where death occurs (at home or elsewhere)
- To have access to information and expertise of whatever kind is necessary
- To have access to any spiritual or emotional support required
- To have access to hospice care in any location, not only in hospital
- To have control over who is present and who shares the end
- To be able to issue advance directives which ensure wishes are respected
- To have time to say goodbye and control over other aspects of timing
- To be able to leave when it is time to go and not to have life prolonged pointlessly.

Terminal care is discussed in Chapter 13.

After death

Following death, relatives usually ask about what will happen to the body. They need explanation and written information about the need for certificates and registration of the death and also how to contact the funeral directors. Funeral directors will also give helpful support and advice to the bereaved relatives.

Bereavement care is covered in Chapter 11.

11

Grief and bereavement

The members of the primary care team are uniquely placed to provide bereavement care. They will often have been involved with the patient and their partner long before the diagnosis of the life-threatening illness was made, seen them through many of its stages, and then cared for them in the final weeks and months. The doctor may well continue as an advisor of the bereaved spouse or close family for years to come. The way in which bereavement support is provided varies from one practice to another.

In bereavement care the roles of the doctor, nurse, social worker, and health visitor are complementary. Voluntary organizations, clergy, and palliative care teams may also be sources of support to the bereaved.

Grief

When does grief start?

Grieving may start even before the diagnosis is confirmed, when the relative senses that the patient they care about is going to die. When the diagnosis is confirmed, no matter how optimistic an outlook is given, most relatives fear the worst but may not mention these fears or grief to anyone.

This concealed grieving may be made even more difficult if for some reason the patient has not been honestly informed of the diagnosis but the relatives are aware. They may have vetoed the patient being told or they may have requested that the patient not be told and so initiated a process of collusion.

Cancer brings its own unique problems. With modern active treatment, patients go into long spells of remission with high hopes of cure, only to have them dashed during each relapse. Hopes rise each time the patient sees specialists who offer radiotherapy or chemotherapy, even though the professionals try to make sure that patients realize that the aims of treatment are palliative.

Patients and relatives both often keep their feelings to themselves in this situation, each wrapped up in their own grief, each fearing that talking it through with each other would hurt the one they love. In this way grief deepens, made worse by partial knowledge, a conspiracy of silence and feelings hidden from the world.

Is grief always normal?

Loss is an integral part of life and grief will be experienced in many forms at different times by each of us. However, we can all be comforted and supported through this difficult time. Members of the primary care team are in a good position to help because their knowledge and communication skills enable them to replace fear with knowledge.

Can grief be harmful?

It is certainly important for general practitioners to always consider whether a patient has features of clinical depression rather than grieving. There is also evidence that the bereaved have an increase incidence in anxiety, alcohol use, consumption of prescribed medication, and suicides. Studies of physical morbidity after bereavement are inconclusive. However, it is thought that widowers have a higher risk of developing a serious illness in the first year of bereavement.

Features of normal grief

An understanding of bereavement theories is useful if we are to improve the patient care and understanding. The various theories surrounding grief and mourning are beyond the scope of this book and further details can be found in the bibliography. Theories, however, have practical implications for practice.

The bereaved generally do not move from one emotional stage of grieving to the next over weeks or months. Grieving responses may include shock, anger, denial, sadness, anxiety, and distress. However, we now know that the bereaved person normally oscillates from time to time between two different orientations, loss and restoration.

Behaviour which is loss orientated involves facing grief, and the distress of grief work. When the bereaved are focusing on loss orientation, they are preoccupied with the thoughts of the dead person, crying over the death, visiting the grave.

The other psychological stance is restoration-orientated behaviour, which includes avoidance, denial, being involved in other things, and

LIVERPOOL JOHN MOORES UNIVERSITY
LEARNING & INFORMATION SERVICES

suppressing the grief. Here the bereaved are distancing themselves from painful thoughts by work or play and involving themselves in new experiences. Concentration entirely on one orientation to the exclusion of the other signifies an abnormal grief. For instance, prolonged preoccupation with the loss would equate to chronic grief. Persistent restoration without loss behaviour would signal delayed or absent grief.

Another approach to grief is based on the bereaved's need to talk about the deceased in an attempt to create a story that they can integrate into their ongoing lives. This narrative approach allows for the creation of a new identity that includes a persistent memory of the deceased. The narrative approach has important implications for bereavement support as it emphasizes the therapeutic value in listening to the bereaved person's story.

Abnormal grief

There is much debate in the literature about the precise nature of abnormal grieving and this probably reflects a professional concern about the medicalization of grief. Normal grieving is a self-limiting process that, however distressing in terms of feelings of sadness, longing for the deceased person, and somatic complaints, does resolve with subsequent recovery. Features of normal grieving overlap those of psychiatric disorder, depression, anxiety, post-traumatic stress disorder, substance abuse, and bereavement disorders.

In addition to the psychological bereavement theories, cultural influences also form a crucial part of the context of bereavement.

Bereavement disorders include the following:

- Absent grief—where individuals show no evidence of the emotion of grief developing despite the reality of the death.

- Delayed grief—presents initially like absent grief. However, this avoidance is a conscious effort and the full emotions of grief are eventually expressed after a particular trigger. The trigger may be a seemingly innocuous loss following the bereavement.

- Chronic grief—the normal emotions of grief persist without any reduction over time. This most often occurs in highly dependent relationships.

The difficulty in defining abnormal grief is complicated by the influence of culturally determined mourning practices. The overlap with syndromes of clinical depression may be difficult to separate out from the grief process.

Factors affecting grief outcome

The challenge of good palliative care involves planning and anticipation as far as is possible. No one is ever the same again after they have lost someone they love. Grief can change both individuals and families. Some people turn to alcohol or drugs, but many more become more mature and responsible. We need to remember that death is not always an unwelcome blow. Not all change is destructive, but we sometimes overlook this in our society, which often seeks to deny the creative powers, which can be unleashed as a result of loss, whether by death or disability.

Family doctors may well have a good knowledge of the carer's background and should heed their intuition if they feel the person is going to be at risk. Doctors need to remember the factors predisposing to abnormal grief and try to identify those who may need closer monitoring and support.

◆ Time to prepare for the deceased's death

Sudden unexpected death is usually a devastating loss. On the other hand, when someone can be helped to come to terms with an expected death, there will still be sadness but it will not usually be so prolonged or destructive if they were supported, kept informed, and shown how to share in the care.

However, it must not be assumed that the longer a patient knows that the death of a loved one is inevitable, the easier it will be. Paradoxically, a very protracted death can also produce bereavement problems.

◆ Age

Age can be a factor in Western society. Loss of a partner at a young age carries more of a risk for women than at an older age.

◆ The nature of the relationship

Those with a particularly ambivalent relationship are more likely to have problems. This may be due to a feeling of guilt, because the death has not only robbed them of the person who was important to them but also removed the chance for resolution of unfinished emotional business.

It has already been stated that not everyone regards death as a disaster. For some it may be a release, a new freedom. For many others it can be a reminder of a relationship that could have been better had both parties worked harder at it and now that opportunity has passed forever.

◆ Stigmatized deaths

Stigmatized death increases the distress for the bereaved. Death by suicide or AIDs provides vivid examples.

◆ Opportunity to care for the patient

Providing carers feel supported themselves and their own needs recognized, they can benefit from having shared in the physical care of the patient. Increasing numbers of patients are dying in hospitals, hospices, and nursing homes, and relatives become increasingly unfamiliar with caring for a dying person at home. One of the challenges for the primary care team is the assessment of what elements of care the family could provide, how the carers can be instructed and guided, and how they should be encouraged and supported in providing care.

◆ Relatives' perception of support

Those who do not feel supported or understood often suffer bad grief reactions, irrespective of how much help they may in fact have received. It is important for the primary care team to make an assessment of how the relatives perceive their support. In drawing a genogram, a superficial inspection may give the impression that a relative is well supported by brothers, sisters, sons, daughters, and grandchildren. However, in questioning the relative, it may be that they find they are unable to accept help or the immediate family is unable to give time from work to help.

◆ Unresolved previous grief

Grief reactions are cumulative. Someone who has not yet 'got over' a bereavement of a year or two before is at risk of further grief problems. The family doctor may be well placed to know of previous losses and appreciate the added burden the new one will bring. Some people only begin to grieve for the previous loss when they start to grieve for the latest one.

◆ Poor socio-economic circumstances

In bereavement, as in so many clinical conditions, people from poor socio-economic circumstances often fare badly.

Providing bereavement support: guidelines for general practitioners

General practitioners need to become more involved in bereavement care. At one level there is a need to raise general awareness of bereavement issues, to train primary health care teams in bereavement care, and to use audit and practice guidelines to improve care of the bereaved.

Specific guidelines may address the following issues:

◆ Use an efficient means of notifying the practice team of the death of a patient. This avoids the embarrassing error of a member of the team visiting a patient's home in ignorance that death has occurred the previous day.

◆ Keep a record of the death in the bereaved's notes.

◆ A personal letter of condolence may be appropriate in some circumstances.

◆ Provide written information about grief, the local support services available, and practical advice.

◆ A bereavement visit soon after death is important as a demonstration of respect and affection for someone you may have known and cared for, perhaps for years.

◆ Make an assessment visit or appointment at 3–6 months after death to find out how the bereaved person is coping. This is a time when friends and family may feel that the bereaved person has 'got over it', when in fact they are most in need of a listening ear.

◆ Use risk assessment in planning bereavement follow-up care.

◆ Some practices may offer professional bereavement counselling within the practice, perhaps involving a counsellor, psychologist, or social worker.

Bereavement counselling and therapy

General practitioners may wish to use their counselling skills in providing bereavement counselling or they may work with a counsellor or psychologist in the practice.

Generally, much bereavement counselling has been based on the concept of grief work. This entails listening to the bereaved person work through the reality of the loss and describing the pain of grief. Once this difficult work has been carried out, the person can begin to adjust to life without their loved one. At a later time they may achieve resolution from grief by emotionally incorporating the deceased into their life and finding they have the strength to take up new interests and become involved once more in a future.

For further details of this grief work please refer to the bibliography.

Bereavement support

The most common types of service offered to bereaved people are individual interviews, group sessions, and telephone contacts. Individual bereavement counselling has been shown to be most effective for those assessed as at risk, especially when the bereaved perceived their families to be unhelpful.

Others have found the use of trained bereavement volunteers from specialist palliative care services helpful and have reduced the use of GP services.

Issues for the general practice include involving the carers in and around the time of death. Once someone has died, the different carers want to spend different amounts of time with the body and there is no right amount of time. Some carers, particularly those who have been involved in the physical care of the dead person, may appreciate being asked if they would like to help wash and prepare the body. Since a death at home is more unusual, few carers will have any previous experience of this. They may be unaware that they can take their time over saying goodbye and the doctor does not have to be called in the middle of the night if he has been visiting the patient recently and that other relatives or friends may be called to make their farewells before the funeral director removes the body.

In meeting the needs for bereaved people, the general practitioner needs to remember young children, the frail elderly, and those with learning disabilities, who may be excluded from contact in the hope that this will protect them from distress. It is important to involve children so that they can say goodbye. Children need permission to see the body of the deceased if they wish, to have the choice of attending the funeral, and to have their questions answered. Many young, bereaved children have questions about the meaning of terms such as cancer, chemotherapy, and radiotherapy. They may want explanations about what happens to a person's body after death. They need time to explore these and many other issues.

We need a range of different services available to help bereaved people who can then choose what they feel is most appropriate for them. Some, for instance, might want one-to-one support, whereas others feel more comfortable in a group; others may prefer telephone contact.

Clear, written information is usually welcomed, particularly if this includes a list of local and national support groups. It is crucially important that primary care teams, specialist palliative care services, and voluntary bereavement services have close links so that care can be co-ordinated.

Conclusion

Primary care teams need to evolve a practice policy towards bereavement support involving all members of the team. Doctors need to remember that the bereaved that are most in need of help may not come to the doctor of their own accord. There needs to be some system of inviting them or contacting them to assess how they are getting on. Doctors need to be familiar with the local voluntary bereavement counselling services and which patients might benefit from their services. In giving support, do not rush into prescribing sedation or antidepressants. Above all, there is a need to have a flexible approach that respects the experience and wishes of the bereaved.

12

Professional stress in palliative care

Palliative care is a challenging specialty. Doctors and nurses need to be aware of the potential emotional costs to themselves in working with patients who are dying. This short chapter outlines some of the areas in palliative care that can cause stress, and discusses ways to minimize stress and avoid burnout.

Complaints

Unsatisfactory communication lies at the heart of many of the stresses experienced by general practitioners and community nurses. Patients or, more commonly, their relatives may complain about the care they have received. Such complaints need to be considered carefully and most practices have developed a local complaints procedure.

Bereaved relatives may focus their anger on the general practitioner, blaming her for delays in diagnosis or inadequate pain control. The relative needs to have a chance to talk about his complaint and to have his concerns listened to in a sensitive way. This may be difficult for the general practitioner, particularly if she feels guilty or angry herself. If mistakes have been made, the sooner these are acknowledged and apologized for, the better. Unfortunately, some doctors still adopt an approach advocated by some car insurance companies, which advise their clients never to admit blame. To say 'I am sorry' is probably the best way of defusing anger if a mistake has been made. Many relatives only want an explanation and an apology for what they perceive as inadequate care.

On the other hand, anger is often part of the grieving process and in this context it is not helpful for relatives to receive defensive letters from the professionals. These relatives need counselling and support, not lawyers and the courts.

Some complaints are generated by professionals. It is all too easy, in the heat of the moment, for a junior hospital doctor to say to a patient 'If only you had been referred earlier'. A patient or relative then can lose confidence in the professional team. If doctors or nurses have reservations about their colleague's management, these should be discussed with the professional concerned, not in front of the patient or relative. One never enhances one's own reputation by denigrating others, whether it is another doctor, community nurse, or Macmillan nurse.

Handling uncertainty

Much of palliative care is uncertain; for instance, prognosis is difficult to predict. Working in the community is often chaotic. There are endless interruptions, unplanned visits, emergencies, and breakdowns in communication which all go towards increasing uncertainty. Decisions have to be made with inadequate information in an environment where advice from colleagues may be conflicting. Doctors need to be able to acknowledge this uncertainty, to work flexibly, and to share the uncertainty with colleagues and the patient and relatives. If the professionals and the patient and family can understand and accept this uncertainty from the outset, then care becomes easier. The alternative is to create unrealistic expectations in the patient and family, leading to disenchantment and anger when these expectations are not fulfilled. It is hard work sitting, listening to patients and helping them to lower their expectations to realistic levels.

The evidence-based medicine movement can foster a false belief that there are always logical solutions to the problems encountered in palliative care. However, although our practice must be informed by the best evidence and research, intuition and experience play an important part in our professional judgements.

Perhaps the biggest challenge facing doctors and nurses is to involve the patient and family in decision making as equal partners in care. Accepting their treatment choices may not be comfortable for the doctor or nurse but it is a powerful sign of respect for the patient.

Ethical dilemmas

As we have seen, ethical dilemmas are heightened at the end of life. The struggle to do the right thing is often stressful. Colleagues can provide useful sounding boards to discuss the problems. Sometimes it is helpful to have a family meeting to include the key team members to try to reach a moral decision. Moral consensus can be hard to achieve, particularly when this area of work is given such a high media profile.

Time management

Lack of time is often cited as a source of stress. Clinical workload can present a threat to the professional's personal life. Achieving a healthy balance between work and home is often difficult. Primary care now embraces formidable managerial responsibilities, which can lead to great stress for clinicians with little or no training to meet these demands. Doctors and nurses need the support of efficient secretarial and administrative staff if they are to organize their work effectively. Sometimes we need to learn to say 'no', when we are invited to attend yet another futile meeting.

The emotional costs of caring

In palliative care, professionals are often involved in difficult emotional conversations with dying patients. Such caring involves a sharing of the patient's distress and is emotionally exhausting for the doctor or nurse. Feelings of failure or helplessness are common in this area of care. Prolonged suffering that is difficult to relieve presents a particular challenge. We need to create a work environment that acknowledges this burden and gives professionals an opportunity to express and share their distress. Doctors and nurses need to know what specialist palliative care resources are available and how to access them.

Keeping up to date

When professionals feel inadequate due to a lack of knowledge, this can be stressful.

Asking for help from specialist palliative care teams may seem a simple solution. However, it is often the most knowledgeable doctors who contact others to discuss a case and the doctors and nurses who most need help who are reluctant to seek it. Specialists can help here by providing education programmes and by never seeming critical of colleagues who seek help. Specialist teams exist to facilitate and enable primary care teams to provide care, not to take over care or to leave colleagues feeling deskilled.

Teamwork

No individual can possibly meet all the needs of the dying patient and his family. Thus, multidisciplinary team working lies at the heart of palliative care. Working in teams inevitably creates conflicts. These need addressing sooner rather than later.

If team members have a clear idea of their roles and the goals of care then many problems are resolved.

Palliative care is one specialty where the roles of doctor and nurse may overlap. This creates a potential for misunderstanding and conflict. For example, in a secure healthy team a nurse may question a doctor's decision and this may lead to a better decision in the patient's care. Unfortunately, the identical situation may be perceived by a vulnerable doctor as criticism and result in conflict and hardening of attitudes.

Perhaps one of the most important parts of teamwork is effective leadership, which encourages a culture where every member of the team knows they are valued and respected.

Home and work

Doctors and nurses need to find ways of balancing their work with their family life. Outside interests, hobbies, and holidays are essential if professionals are to enjoy a healthy life. Team members who always work late need just as much support and attention as those who are frequently absent with minor illnesses. Teams can experience burnout as well as individuals.

We need to develop ways of caring for our colleagues with as much sensitivity as we do for our patients.

Clinical supervision and mentoring

These forms of professional support are most developed in the nursing and social work disciplines. However, similar models may well have a role in helping to support medical staff. Peer appraisal should be educative and supportive rather than threatening. Professionals working in palliative care should have the choice to discuss their professional practice with a colleague in a structured way if they wish. Such discussions can identify areas where practice is going well and others where improvements could be made.

13

The final days:
terminal care at home

Diagnosing the terminal phase

The doctor has an important role in establishing that the patient is in the terminal phase of the illness. This is not always straightforward. Diagnosing the terminal phase is a clinical skill. The patient is generally weak and spends much of the day in bed. He might be drowsy and sometimes disorientated and confused. The patient is not interested in food and often has difficulty swallowing both solids and liquids.

The most important clue to the fact that the patient is entering the terminal stage is the rate of physical deterioration. At this stage the patient is visibly weaker day by day. This change in the progression of the illness is often more apparent to relatives and nurses than the doctor. Doctors need to listen to the nursing view as to whether the patient is in the terminal phase because their intuitions are generally right.

The signs that the patient is dying are a decreased body temperature with cold peripheries, respiration becomes shallower and Cheyne–Stokes respiration may be observed. The blood pressure falls, colour fades, and the patient has a weak, rapid, thready pulse.

The aims of care in the terminal phase are to enable the patient to die with dignity, thus there is no place for further investigations or treatments that carry harmful side-effects. It is a time when it is important to review care from the perspective of the patient, and while the care remains centred on the patient, it is important at this stage to review the medication, the nursing care, and the care of the relatives.

Review medication

The key points to caring in this phase are to continue only the essential drugs and discontinue all the others. The essential drugs that need to be reviewed are analgesics, sedatives, and possibly anticonvulsants. The general practitioner is in a good position to forewarn the relatives that a time will come when non-essential medication will have to be discontinued, thus making it easier to do so at a later date.

Examples of non-essential drugs that may be discontinued include iron, vitamins, cardiac drugs, hypoglycaemic and anti-hypertensive agents, diuretics, potassium supplements, long-term antibiotics, antidepressants, and H2 antagonists.

Route of administration

The oral route may no longer be feasible and the use of the subcutaneous syringe driver has enabled many patients to remain at home while receiving appropriate medication. Again, the general practitioner can prepare the patient and relatives for this at an earlier time. Drugs commonly used in the syringe driver in this phase include diamorphine for pain, midazolam as the sedative of choice, and an antiemetic such as methotrimeprazine or haloperidol. Hyoscine butylbromide may be used to control excessive secretions.

Anticipating problems is the hallmark of the skilled clinician. At this stage, it is important to remember to supply drugs at home, which might be necessary for breakthrough pain, agitation, or noisy secretions.

Pain

Always assume that there may be breakthrough pain and plan accordingly. The dose of an opioid for such events should be one-sixth of the total daily opioid intake whether they are on morphine solution every 4 hours or subcutaneous by syringe driver. The syringe driver booster button is not a form of patient-controlled analgesia. Pressing the button only delivers a minute dose, which is totally inadequate for pain relief.

Patients with bone pain may require continuation of their non-steroidal anti-inflammatory drugs (NSAIDs), which may be conveniently given in either suppository form, naproxen 500 milligrams twice a day, or in some cases by subcutaneous infusion ketorolac 30–60 milligrams over 24 hours.

Restlessness

This should not be an inevitable feature of the final days. When it does occur, it is important to exclude straightforward causes such as pain, a full bladder, or a pressure sore. If there is no easily reversible factor, the patient should be given midazolam in the syringe driver in a dose of 30–60 milligrams over 24 hours with breakthrough midazolam supplied, which can be given by subcutaneous injection. Methotrimeprazine in a dose of 50–150 milligrams over 24 hours in the syringe driver is an effective alternative and particularly useful if vomiting is also a problem.

Noisy secretions

The death rattle of noisy secretions is extremely distressing for the relatives, but not for the patient. Explain that the patient will not be distressed and warn the relatives that it may occur and that drugs will be given to help to control it.

Hyoscine butylbromide is preferable to the hydrobromide and is given at a 20 milligrams stat subcutaneous injection and between 20 and 60 milligrams over 24 hours in the syringe driver. It is equally as effective in drying secretions as hyoscine hydrobromide but tends to cause less mental confusion.

Convulsions

These can be controlled either with subcutaneous midazolam 5–10 milligrams subcutaneous stat or 1 milligrams per minute intravenously or 30–60 milligrams over 24 hours in the syringe driver or rectal diazepam solution 20 milligrams pr, usually effective in 10–15 minutes.

An alternative, if there is cerebral irritation due to brain metastases, is phenobarbitone intramuscular injections 100–200 milligrams stat or a subcutaneous aqueous solution infusion 400–800 milligrams over 24 hours in a separate syringe driver.

Haemorrhage

Massive haemorrhage is a particularly traumatic event in the terminal stage. The doctor needs to spend time with patients and relatives assessing their degree of anxiety and offering admission to hospice or hospital if this is requested.

At home there should be a supply of dark-coloured towels to minimize the frightening appearance of the blood. The doctor should leave supplies of diamorphine and midazolam, which can be given to sedate the patient.

In an opioid naïve patient diamorphine 10 milligrams and midazolam 10 milligrams may be given together either intravenously or subcutaneously. In a patient who is already receiving diamorphine via the syringe driver, one-third of the daily dose should be given by injection.

Relatives and staff will need time after the event to talk of their distress. Massive haemorrhage is usually so sudden that there is no time to give drugs and this can add to the distress of the carers and nurses.

Dyspnoea

Terminal dyspnoea is best controlled with a combination of opioids and midazolam.

In an opioid naïve patient, diamorphine 10 milligrams over 24 hours may be given subcutaneously using the syringe driver. If this fails to relieve the distress then midazolam 10 milligrams over 24 hours may be added to the driver or single subcutaneous injections of 1.25–2.5 milligrams may be administered.

Vomiting

Methotrimeprazine is particularly useful for treating vomiting in the terminal phase, as its sedative effect is often beneficial. It may be used as a single injection at night of 12.5–25 milligrams or in the syringe driver 25–150 milligrams subcutaneously over 24 hours.

Other drugs which may be helpful are cyclizine 150 milligrams over 24 hours and haloperidol 5 milligrams over 24 hours. These should be administered subcutaneously using the syringe driver.

Drugs in the bag

It is helpful for doctors to have a supply of the following drugs in their bag for the care of the patient who is dying at home (see Appendix 3).

+ Diamorphine
+ Dexamethasone
+ Hyoscine butylbromide
+ Midazolam
+ Diazepam rectal
+ Haloperidol
+ Methotrimeprazine

Review the nursing care

The key member of the nursing team at this stage is the district or community nurse who will liaise with specialist nurses such as Macmillan nurses and Marie Curie nurses and also with the general practitioner and social services.

The co-ordinating role is a key one to ensure that there is the right balance between the patient receiving the appropriate advice and review and respecting the privacy of the patient at home.

Mouth care

Candidiasis can continue to be a problem to the end of life. The family and carers can be taught how to continue with mouth care, with iced drinks and lollipop sponges to moisten the mouth. Keeping the mouth moist and fresh requires mouth care at least hourly if candidiasis is a problem.

Meticulous mouth care in the terminal phase will relieve thirst and thus remove the need for intravenous hydration at this stage.

Pressure sore care

When the patient is in the dying phase it is no longer appropriate for frequent turnings to be carried out and it is safe and appropriate for the patient to be left almost undisturbed in the most comfortable position. It is important that the patient has the appropriate mattress and padding to protect heels, elbows, and knees. Skin care is still important.

Bowel care

Bowel care in this end stage is no longer a priority. Oral laxatives can be stopped and rectal treatment only given if the patient is clearly uncomfortable as a result of a loaded rectum.

Bladder care

If the patient is not passing much urine, there is no problem now. If he is passing more than a little, it should be discussed with the patient and the family whether he should be catheterized to save moving him and to maintain care. Catheterization is preferable to sheaths or incontinence pads in maintaining dignity and helping skin care.

The home environment

Every detail of the room needs to be reviewed. Is the bed in the best position for attendants to help the patient? Can the light be dimmed? What are the arrangements made for a night-light? Can the noise be reduced, ventilation improved, extraneous smells reduced? Are there chairs for the family to sit on or sleep in? Is there a table for teacups, mugs, tissues, towels, and pads near at hand?

Review care of the relatives

Ensure relatives are informed and up to date. Relatives may have understood the original diagnosis and treatment but it is important that they are kept up to date with developments, particularly now that the patient is changing on a daily basis. They may have known that the patient is seriously ill and probably that he will die, but that he is actually dying now is often a shock. They should be told explicitly, preferably as a family and, better still, with the doctor and nurse present. Not only do they need to know that we are talking of the final days, but also what will happen during those days. They will need reassurance that morphine is not shortening the patient's life.

Many relatives have not seen a death or touched a body. The doctor needs to explain the colour changes, the cooling of the extremities, Cheyne–Stoke respiration, the rattle of secretions, and confusion—everything that they may observe and worry about and of which they are possibly too embarrassed and frightened to speak.

Each member of the family needs to be informed of the situation and the new care plan and priorities negotiated with them: which drugs have been discontinued and why; which are now more important than ever; why and how they will be given; what might happen and the responses that the doctor and nurse have planned together.

Remember that, for many, this is a totally new experience for which they feel unprepared and unskilled. They need skilled, professional support, which does not mean taking over care but rather enabling them to contribute to the caring. One well-recognized factor in grief reactions of relatives is the feeling that they were not able or permitted to help in the patient's care. At home this need never happen. Relatives can be taught mouth care, sponging and talcing, preparing crushed ice, and so on. For those who cannot bear to touch the patient, they can do some of the shopping or man the telephone.

Support of the relatives is a challenge for the palliative care team because each member of the family displays different faces of grief. Some are quiet and others angry, some ask questions, while others pretend they don't want to know. Some suspect the others but there is nearly always one who either blames the rest or takes command.

Listening to the relatives will enable the doctor to have a chance to defuse tensions and prevent hostilities. He can demonstrate how each relative can contribute and actually grow through this experience. Relatives may have fears if dying is prolonged and will need reassurance that we are neither hastening death nor prolonging suffering but all working together to maintain the dignity of the dying patient

Emergency routine

The family may have been telephoning the surgery in the past, but when the patient dies no one can find the telephone number! It is important that the family knows clearly how to access the doctor on call, the district nurse or community nurse and to have telephone numbers available. It may be relevant to also have the number of their local minister, priest, or rabbi if this is something they have indicated is important.

Professional support

Whilst the general practitioner and district nurses are the key professional players at this phase of care, it is important to remember that the specialist multidisciplinary palliative care team are also available for advice and help. This could be by telephone, for domiciliary visits, or to provide in-patient support.

Another important contribution that the specialists can make is that, when there has been a difficult death, it is often helpful to review the case in a discussion with the professionals involved, perhaps facilitated by one of the specialist palliative care team.

One of the most powerful ways of giving support to patients and their families is for the general practitioner and district nurse to continue to visit the dying patient at home. Even though the doctor may not feel he is contributing much at this stage it is always worthwhile to continue to visit. These visits need to be co-ordinated with the nurses and other members of the primary care team, to cause the minimum disruption to the family.

Appendix 1

Bibliography

Comprehensive reference books on palliative medicine

Doyle, D., Hanks, G. W., and MacDonald, N. (1997). *Oxford textbook of palliative medicine* (2nd edn). Oxford University Press, Oxford.

Sims, R. and Moss, V. A. (1995). *Palliative care for people with AIDS*. Edward Arnold, London.

Woodruff, R. (1999). *Palliative medicine: symptomatic and supportive care for patients with advanced cancer and AIDS* (3rd edn). Oxford University Press, Oxford.

Communication and ethics issues

Buckman, R. (1988). *I don't know what to say—how to help and support someone who is dying*. Macmillan, London.

Buckman, R. (1993). *How to break bad news—a guide for healthcare professionals*. Macmillan Medical, London.

Jeffrey, D. (1993). *There is nothing more I can do*. Patten Press, Penzance.

Myerscough, P. R. and Ford, M. (1996). *Talking with patients—keys to good communication* (3rd edn). Oxford University Press, Oxford.

Randall, F. and Downie, R. S. (1999). *Palliative care ethics—a companion for all specialties* (2nd edn). Oxford University Press, Oxford.

Cultural issues

Neuberger, J. (1987). *Caring for dying people of different faiths*. Lisa Sainsbury Foundation, Surrey/Austin Cornish Publishers.

Bereavement

Ainsworth-Smith, I. and Speck, P. (1983). *Letting go*. SPCK, London.

Parkes, C. M. (1986). *Bereavement: studies of grief in adult life*. Tavistock Publications, New York.

Speck, P. (1978). *Loss and grief in medicine*. Ballière Tindall, London.

Walter, T. (1994). *The revival of death*. Routledge, London.

Worden, J. W. (1991). *Grief counselling and grief therapy* (2nd edn). Tavistock Publications, London.

Information for patients

Asthma: the National Asthma Campaign publishes a large number of leaflets and booklets on every aspect of asthma for patients (adults and children), carers, and professionals. Write to National Asthma Campaign, Asthma Enterprises Limited, Providence House, Providence Place, London N1 0NT, or fax: 020-7704-0740.

BACUP publications: a wide range of useful up-to-date publications on individual cancers and their treatments—for patients and professionals. Available from 121–123 Charterhouse Street, London, EC1M 6AA.

Chest, heart and stroke, Scotland Publications. Order free booklets from 65 North Castle Street, Edinburgh, EH2 3LT.

The cancer guide: information for people with cancer and those who care (1997). Macmillan Cancer Relief, London.

Helping the relatives and carers

Burton, L. (1974). *Care of the child facing death*. Routledge and Paul, London.

Cassidy, S. (1988). *Sharing the darkness*. Darton, Longman and Todd, London.

Doyle, D. (1994). *Caring for a dying relative*. Oxford University Press, Oxford.

Stedeford, A. (1994). *Facing death; patients, families and professionals*. Sobell Publications, Oxford.

'Which' guide: *Understanding cancer* (1986). Consumers Association Publishers, London.

Hospices and hospice care

Doyle, D. (1999). *The platform ticket: memories and musings of a hospice doctor*. Pentland Press, Durham.

Lewis, M. (1992). *Tears and smiles*. Michael O'Mara Books, London.

Books for and about children

Goldman, A. (1998). *Care of the dying child* (rev. edn). Oxford University Press, Oxford.

Krementz, J. (1983). *How it feels when a parent dies*. Victor Gollancz, London.

Rando, T. (1986). *Parental loss of a child*. Research Press, Champaign, Illinois.

Snell, N. (1987). *Emma's cat dies*. Hamish Hamilton, London.

Appendix 2

Useful addresses

Bereavement

Child Bereavement Trust
Harleyford Estate
Henley Road
Marlow SL7 2DX

Tel. 01628 488101

The Trust provides resources and information for bereaved families and the professionals who care for them. It also provides training and support for professionals to enable them to meet the needs of grieving families.

Child Death Helpline
Bereavement Services Department
Great Ormond Street Hospital NHS Trust
London WC1N 3JH

Tel. 020 7813 8551

The Child Death Helpline is operated from Great Ormond Street and the Alder Hey Children's Hospital. It is staffed by bereaved parents and it is a confidential helpline for anyone affected by the death of a child.

Compassionate Friends
53 North Street
Bristol BS3 1EN

Tel. 0117 966 5202

A nationwide organization of bereaved parents offering friendship and understanding to other bereaved parents after the death of a son or daughter from any cause whatsoever. Personal and group support. Quarterly newsletter, postal library, and range of leaflets. Support for bereaved siblings and grandparents. Befriending rather than counselling.

Cruse Bereavement Care
Cruse House
126 Sheen Road
Richmond
Surrey TW9 1UR

Tel. 020 8332 7227

Offers free bereavement counselling and support to anyone who has been bereaved, visiting them in their own home. Has an extensive publications list along with useful leaflets and newsletters. Offers social contact with specialist services to various bereaved groups.

Jewish Bereavement Counselling Service
PO Box 6748
London N3 3BX

Tel. 020 8349 0839

Counselling and support for all members of the family who have been bereaved, provided by trained voluntary counsellors who are professionally supervised.

Lesbian and Gay Bereavement Project
AIDS Education Unit
Vaughan M Williams Centre
Colindale Hospital
London NW9 5GH

Tel. 020 8200 0511

Helpline 020 8455 8894
(19:00 to midnight daily)

The project offers advice, support, and counselling to bereaved gay men and lesbians, their families and friends. They also educate professional and voluntary carers within the community in same-sex groups.

NAFSIYAT
Intercultural Therapy Centre
278 Seven Sisters Road
Finsbury Park
London N4 2HY

Tel. 020 7263 4130

Nafsiyat is a voluntary organization providing a psychotherapeutic service to people from black and ethnic minorities and from racially mixed relationships. It provides a low-cost service including bereavement counselling to individuals, couples, families, and groups. As well as self-referrals, health and social service contacts are received.

National Association of Bereavement Services
20 Norton Folgate
London E1 6DB

Tel. 020 7247 1080

Refers bereaved people to their appropriate local service. Promotes networking, training, and professional standards. Publishes National Directory of Bereavement and Loss Services.

Winston's Wish
Gloucestershire Royal Hospital
Great Western Road
Gloucester GL1 3NN

Tel. 01452 394377

This grief support programme provides free a service for bereaved children and their families in Gloucestershire. Information about resources and national training workshops are available on request. Based on experience of working with over 1000 children and their families, Winston's Wish offers a comprehensive training and consultancy package for professionals who wish to develop similar services in other areas.

Cancer information

CancerBACUP
3 Bath Place
Rivington Street
London EC2A 3JR

Tel. 020 7696 9003
Helpline 0800 181199

CancerBACUP provides a national telephone and letter information service on all aspects of cancer for people with cancer, their families and friends. Face-to-face counselling is provided in London (020 7696 9000) and Glasgow (0141 553 1553).

CancerLink
11–21 Northdown Street
London N1 9BN

Tel. 020 7833 2818
Helpline 0800 132905

Freephone Asian Cancer Information in Bengali, Hindi, Punjabi, Urdu, and English: 0800 590415.

Freephone MAC Helpline for young people affected by cancer: 0800 591028.

CancerLink offers emotional support and information on all aspects of cancer in response to telephone and letter enquiries from people affected by cancer, their families, friends, and other professionals working with them. Acts as a resource to cancer support and self-help groups and individual supporters throughout the UK and produces a range of publications on emotional and practical issues.

Cancer Black Care
16 Dalston Lane
London E8 3AZ

Helpline 020 7249 1097

Offers information and advice and addresses the cultural and emotional needs of black people affected by cancer, as well as their families and friends. Also offers advocacy, interpretation, and a training and cultural awareness programme for health professionals.

Irish Cancer Society
5 Northumberland Road
Dublin 4
Ireland

Tel. 010 353 1 668 1855
Helpline 1 8000 200700

A charity whose services include a Cancer Helpline, night-nursing service, professional and public information, home care nurses, oncology nurse counsellors, patient support groups, research, professional educational programmes, and anti-smoking activities.

Macmillan Information Line
2nd Floor, Angel Walk
Hammersmith
London W6 9HX

Helpline 0845 601 6161

A nationally available telephone information service for people with cancer, their families, friends, and carers. Provides callers with information on Macmillan services and activities, as well as giving details of other cancer organizations and support agencies when appropriate. Macmillan leaflets and publications are also available to callers in support of their enquiry.

The National Cancer Alliance
PO Box 579
Oxford OX4 1LB

Helpline 01865 793566

The NCA is an alliance of patients, carers, and health professionals working together to improve the treatment and care of all cancer patients in Britain. It aims to ensure that high-quality treatment is available to all who need it.

Tak Tent Cancer Support—Scotland
Block 20 Western Court
off University Avenue, 100 University Place
Glasgow G12 6SQ

Helpline 0141 211 1932

Offers emotional support and information on cancers and treatment. Has support groups throughout Scotland, and a resource/drop-in centre. The youth project offers support to those 16–25-year-olds who are patients or relatives.

The Tenovus Cancer Information Centre
College Buildings
Courtenay Road
Splott
Cardiff CF1 1SA

Helpline 0800 526527

Written and verbal information on all aspects of cancer available free of charge for patients and their families. Helpline staffed by nurses, counsellors, and social workers. Individual counselling face to face or via the telephone. Support nurses available at Velindre, Llandough, Cardiff, and Wrexham hospitals.

Carers National Association
20–25 Glasshouse Yard
London EC1A 4JS

Helpline 0345 573369

The organization aims to encourage carers to recognize their own needs, and to provide support. There is an information team for professionals as well as a carers' advice and information team. The organization brings carers' concerns to the attention of government.

ACT Association for Children with life-threatening or terminal conditions and their families
65 St Michael's Hill
Bristol BS2 8OZ

Tel. 0117 922 1556

A national resource and information service for families and health care professionals involved in caring for children with life-threatening and terminal illness. The organization is concerned with representing the needs of children and families throughout the UK. ACTS has a multidisciplinary membership.

Sargent Cancer Care for Children
14 Abingdon Road
London W8 6AF

Helpline 020 7656 5100

Counselling and practical support provided by Sargent social workers at major hospitals. Cash grants for extra expenses, e.g. travel to hospitals, heating bills, clothing, etc. Grants for treats (books, games) and holidays. Holiday homes in Scotland and Northern Ireland. Application through any hospital social worker if under 21 years of age.

Complementary Cancer Care
Programme
The Royal London Homeopathic
Hospital NHS Trust
Great Ormond Street
London WC1N 3HR

Tel. 020 7837 8833

Offers a programme of homeopathy
and other complementary therapies to
support well-being and quality of life
which may be used in conjunction with
conventional cancer treatments. Referrals via the patient's GP.

Non-cancer illnesses

National AIDS Helpline
PO Box 5000
Glasgow G12 8BR

Tel. 0141 357 1774
Helpline 0800 567123

This is a national phone line offering
confidential advice, information, and
referrals on any aspect of HIV/AIDS to
anyone. All calls are taken by trained
and paid staff. Ethnic language services
available: Bengali, Punjabi, Gujerati,
Urdu, Hindi, Arabic, Cantonese, Welsh.

The Terrence Higgins Trust
52–54 Gray's Inn Road
London WC1X 8JU

Helpline 020 7242 1010

Provides information, advice, and help
to all those concerned about AIDS and
HIV infection. Practical help includes
'buddies' for people with AIDS in the
London area; welfare, housing, and legal
advice; counselling; support groups.

The Naz Project (London)
Palingswick House
241 King Street
London W6 9LP

Tel. 020 8741 1879

Sexual health and HIV and AIDS education, prevention, and support services

for the South Asian, Middle Eastern,
and North African communities.
Befriending service for people living
with HIV and AIDS. Support groups for
people affected and for carers.

Alzheimer's Society
Gordon House
10 Greencoat Place
London SW1P 1PH

Tel. 020 7306 0606

The Society is the leading care and
research charity for people with dementia. It provides information and education, support for carers, and quality day
and home care. It funds medical and
scientific research and campaigns for
improved health and social services
and greater public understanding of
dementia.

Lymphoedema Support Network
St Luke's Crypt
Sydney Street
London SW3 6NH

Tel. 020 7351 4480

The LSN aims to support patients, to
provide information about lymphoedema and its treatment through a
newsletter and other publications, to
work for better resources for treatment,
and to maintain contact with healthcare

professionals working in lymphoedema management. The LSN has over 900 members and is in contact with 26 local support groups.

Motor Neurone Disease Association
PO Box 246
Northampton NN1 2PR

Helpline 0345 626262

Advice and information for people with MND, their families and professionals through national office and Regional Care Advisers. Active branch network of volunteers. Nationwide equipment loan service to people with MND. Limited financial assistance. Basic and professional leaflets available.

Multiple Sclerosis Society
25 Effie Road
Fulham
London SW6 1EE

Helpline 020 7371 8000

Offers information to people with MS, their friends, carers, and family. Financial assistance and welfare services available; bimonthly journal. Over 360 local branches. Send large, stamped addressed envelope for information.

Parkinson's Disease Society
22 Upper Woburn Place
London WC1H 0RA

Helpline 020 7388 5798

Helps all people with Parkinson's disease, their families and the professionals involved in their care. Main activities are research, welfare information and education, field services and fund raising. There are 230 local branches.

Stroke Association
Stroke House
123–127 Whitecross Street
London EC11Y 8JJ

Tel. 020 7490 7999

Works to prevent strokes and to help those who have suffered strokes, and their families. Provides an advisory service from its London office and from 32 regional centres and produces a wide range of publications. Welfare grants are made through social services or health professionals. Community services, Family Support, and Dysphasic Support help new stroke families. The association can put enquirers in touch with their nearest stroke club.

Chest, Heart and Stroke Association—Scotland
65 Castle Street
Edinburgh 2

Tel. 0131 225 6932

National Asthma Campaign
Asthma Enterprises Limited
Providence House
Providence Place
London N1 0NT

This organization publishes a large number of information leaflets and booklets for patients (adult and children), carers, and professionals on every aspect of asthma.

Holidays

A list of organizations offering holiday accommodation for patients and carers is available from the Hospice Information Service, St Christopher's Hospice, London SE26 6DZ.

Tel. 0181 778 9252. E-mail: his@stchris.ftech.co.uk

Information about hospices and specialist palliative care services

Hospice Information Service
St Christopher's Hospice
51 Lawrie Park Road
Sydenham
London SE26 6DZ
Tel. 020 8778 9252

E-mail: his@stchris.ftech.co.uk

The service provides a world-wide resource.

Help the Hospices
Hospice House
34–44 Britannia Street
London WC1X 9JG
Tel. 020 7278 5668
E-mail: info@helpthehospices.org.uk

Appendix 3:

Useful drugs for the doctor's bag

What a doctor carries in his or her emergency bag usually reflects their personality and place of practice. Sadly, in some areas, the contents may have to be constrained as a security precaution against criminals and addicts. Few drugs used in palliative care will need to be carried by the doctor whose patients all live within a relatively short distance from the surgery or health centre. On the other hand, a doctor serving a widely scattered rural population may have to carry sufficient drugs to deal with a large range of emergencies.

The suggestions here are for drugs that might either be carried or kept readily available in health centres or community hospitals. We stress again that emergencies do occur in palliative care and how well they are managed affects not only the patient but also the morale and confidence of the relatives.

Diamorphine 30 milligram ampoules

It is critically important that the doctor has available a dose of strong opioid to control breakthrough or incident pain. Remember that some patients will be on high doses of opiates and the breakthrough dose needs to be calculated to reflect this (see Chapter 3).

It should go without saying that a supply of transdermal or oral opioids need not be carried for pain crises.

Dexamethasone 4 milligram ampoules

May be required for cerebral oedema, spinal cord compression, or superior vena caval obstruction pending admission and definitive treatment.

Hyoscine butylbromide 20 milligram ampoules

Invaluable for death rattle in drying secretions and for the relief of colic.

Midazolam 10 milligram ampoules

One of the most useful drugs in palliative care, it should be available for agitation, panic attacks, and convulsions.

It is usually given as a bolus subcutaneously but can be given intravenously provided the dose rate does not exceed 1 milligram per minute. It is effective for 3 hours, causes amnesia, but also has the propensity to depress respiration.

The stat dose range is 1.25–10 milligrams subcutaneously, the mean daily dose being 30–60 milligrams subcutaneously in 24 hours.

Diazepam rectal solution 10 milligram tubes

This can be administered by relatives, and is effective within 15 minutes.

Haloperidol 5 milligram ampoules

Haloperidol is a useful antiemetic for drug-induced vomiting and has the added benefit of being a tranquillizer. The antiemetic dose is 1.5–2.5 milligrams.

When given for acute paranoid psychotic episodes 5–10 milligrams may be needed in a single dose. Haloperidol has a long half-life so a single dose may last 24 hours.

Methotrimeprazine 25 milligram ampoules

This phenothiazine is both antiemetic and sedative. In low doses of 6.25–12.5 milligrams it has an antiemetic effect without much sedation. However, if sedation is required then an injection of 25–50 milligrams may be given subcutaneously.

Cyclizine 50 milligram ampoules

This is a useful broad-spectrum antiemetic which is helpful in controlling vomiting due to subacute intestinal obstruction.

Appendix 4

Setting up a syringe driver

There are two syringe drivers in use in palliative care:

- Graseby Model MS 26, which is calibrated in millimetres per day and is the most commonly used in palliative care
- Graseby Model MS 16, which is calibrated in millimetres per hour

Providers of palliative care both in hospital and in the community should evolve a common syringe-driver policy which uses one of the above. Having two different types of syringe drivers available in a practice can lead to drug administration errors.

- The boost button is useful to check the function of the driver and is not a means of giving breakthrough subcutaneous analgesia.
- A 10 ml, 20 ml, or rarely a 30 ml syringe can be used. The commonest size is a 10 ml syringe.
- The syringe-driver setting chosen is the distance the plunger of the syringe will travel in 1 day for the MS26 and in 1 hour for the MS16.
- The speed is set at 48 mm per hour on the MS26 and 2 mm per hour on the MS16.
- The butterfly needle is inserted subcutaneously in the anterior abdominal wall, upper chest wall, or upper arm, and is held in place with adhesive film such as Tegaderm.
- The battery is inserted and the booster button pressed to check function.
- The drugs require changing every 24 hours.
- The patient and relative should be educated to check that the driver is functioning.
- The site of infusion is inspected daily and changed every 3 days, or earlier if any redness is developing.

Troubleshooting

- Cannula blockage—change the cannula
- Leaking tubing—again replace
- Blocked tube due to drug precipitation—review drug combination, consider dilution using larger volume syringe
- Syringe may become dislodged if dropped—reposition
- Battery failure—replace
- Inspect skin site for local irritation—change site
- Remember that syringe pumps are not waterproof —they need disconnecting if the patient is having a shower.

Index